Building Muscle for Beginners

The Complete Blueprint to Building Muscle with Weight Lifting

Baz Thompson

© Copyright 2020 - All rights reserved.

The content contained within this book may not be reproduced, duplicated or transmitted without direct written permission from the author or the publisher.

Under no circumstances will any blame or legal responsibility be held against the publisher, or author, for any damages, reparation, or monetary loss due to the information contained within this book, either directly or indirectly.

Legal Notice:

This book is copyright protected. It is only for personal use. You cannot amend, distribute, sell, use, quote or paraphrase any part, or the content within this book, without the consent of the author or publisher.

Disclaimer Notice:

Please note the information contained within this document is for educational and entertainment purposes only. All effort has been executed to present accurate, up to date, reliable, complete information. No warranties of any kind are declared or implied. Readers acknowledge that the author is not engaged in the rendering of legal, financial, medical or professional advice. The content within this book has been derived from various sources. Please consult a licensed professional before attempting any techniques outlined in this book.

By reading this document, the reader agrees that under no circumstances is the author responsible for any losses, direct or indirect, that are incurred as a result of the use of the information contained within this document, including, but not limited to, errors, omissions, or inaccuracies.

Table of Contents

INTRODUCTION 1

BENEFITS OF LEAN AND HEALTHY MUSCLE BUILDING 5
- *Muscles Help Regulate Blood Sugar Levels* 6
- *Muscles Help Control Body Fat* 6
- *Muscles Give You More Functional Strength* 7
- *Muscles Reduce the Risk of Cancer and Cardiovascular Disease* 7
- *Muscles Strengthen Bones, Ligaments, and Joints* 8
- *Muscle-Building Improves Your Emotional and Mental Health* 8
- *Muscles Lengthen Your Lifespan* 9

CHAPTER 1: AN INTRODUCTION TO BUILDING MUSCLE 11

APPROACHES TO HYPERTROPHY 16
- *The Role of Calories in Building Muscle* 16
- *Clean Bulk vs Dirty Bulk* 18

SHOULD YOU DO CARDIO WHILE BUILDING MUSCLE? 20
- *Addressing Your Body Type* 21
- *Catering to Your Goals* 21
- *Bottom Line* 22

THE IMPORTANCE OF SLEEP AND RECOVERY 22

CHAPTER 2: UNDERSTANDING YOUR BODY TYPE 25

THE THREE MAIN BODY TYPES 26
- *Ectomorph* 27
- *Endomorph* 29
- *Mesomorph* 31

FINAL THOUGHTS 34

CHAPTER 3: NUTRITION 37

THE ROLE OF NUTRITION IN BUILDING MUSCLE 38

- THE VALUE OF PROTEIN 41
  - *Figuring Out the Three Macronutrients........................... 42*
- OF CALORIES AND METABOLISM 47
  - *Figuring Out Your Base Metabolic Rate 48*
  - *Caloric Surplus or Deficit?.. 52*
- STRUCTURING YOUR DIET PLAN AROUND THE THREE MACROS 54
  - *What Should Your Plate Look Like?................................ 55*
  - *Best Food for Carbohydrates 57*
  - *Best Food for Fat.. 58*
  - *Best Food for Protein.. 59*
  - *Top Foods to AVOID at All Costs 60*
- BEST SUPPLEMENTS FOR BODYBUILDERS 62
  - *Whey Protein 64*
  - *Casein Protein... 64*
  - *Weight Gainers... 65*
  - *BCAA (Branched Chain Amino Acids) 65*
  - *Creatine.. 66*
  - *Omega-3 Fatty Acids.. 66*
  - *Caffeine 67*
- THE BEST NUTRITION SECRETS, TIPS, AND TRICKS 67
  - *Prioritize Real Food 68*
  - *Don't Be Afraid of Supplements...................................... 68*
  - *Drink Lots of Water... 69*
  - *Track Your Food Intake... 69*
  - *Plan Your Meals.. 70*
  - *Make Adjustments Whenever Necessary....................... 70*
  - *When Unsure, Eat Meat and Vegetables 71*
  - *Fibrous Carbs Over Sugar 71*
  - *Avoid Alcohol.. 72*
  - *Treat Yourself (Sometimes) 72*
- FINAL THOUGHTS 73

CHAPTER 4: REST AND RECOVERY 75

- THE IMPORTANCE OF REST AND RECOVERY 77
- WHAT IS OVERTRAINING? 79
  - *Signs of Overtraining.. 80*
- THE IMPORTANCE OF SLEEP 81
  - *Understanding the Sleep Cycles...................................... 83*

 Negative Effects of Sleep Deprivation............................ 85
The Importance of "Pre"hab... 86
 Understanding Mobility as a Tool for Injury Prevention . 87
 Active Recovery Days... 90
Best Sleep and Recovery Habits 91
 Track Your Sleep 91
 Stay Away from Blue-Light Devices Late at Night........... 91
 Don't Drink Coffee Beyond 2 PM 92
 Avoid Taking Long Naps During the Day......................... 92
 Force Yourself to Wake Up Earlier 93
 Sleep in a Cool Room 93
 Engage in Cross-Training 94
 Do a Proper Warm-Up and Cool Down During Every Training Session... 94
 Devote at Least 10 Minutes Every Day to Mobility Work 95
 Reduce the Amount of Stress in Your Life........................ 95

CHAPTER 5: TRAINING YOUR MUSCLES................................. 97

Compound vs Isolated Movements 99
Holistic Muscle Building.. 101
The Dangers of Muscle Imbalance 102
 What is Muscle Imbalance? 103
 What are the Symptoms of Muscle Imbalance?............ 103
 How Do You Address Muscle Imbalances?.................... 104
Structuring Your Workout Plan 106
 Push-Pull Movements 107
 Upper Body Exercises... 110
 Core Exercises.. 113
 Lower Body Exercises... 116
 Special Note 120
Incorporating Cardio 120
Using Supersets.. 122
Sample 1-Week Bodybuilding Program................................ 123
 Monday (Push + Core).. 124
 Tuesday (Pull)... 125
 Wednesday (Push)... 125
 Thursday (Active Recovery)... 125
 Friday (Pull + Core).. 125

Saturday (Active Recovery).. 126
Sunday (Rest).. 126

CHAPTER 6: PROGRESSIVE OVERLOAD.............................. 127

WHAT IS PROGRESSIVE OVERLOAD? 128
HOW DOES IT BENEFIT YOUR TRAINING? 130
HOW DOES PROGRESSIVE OVERLOAD WORK? 131
Increase Resistance... 131
Increase Volume (Reps)... 132
Increase the Rate of Work... 132
RULES OF PROGRESSIVE OVERLOAD 133
Always Start with Perfect Form 133
Progressive Overload is Not a Linear Process 134
Strength Gains Decrease Over Time and Increased Ability 135

CHAPTER 7: FINAL TIPS TO REMEMBER 137

DON'T OVERTRAIN 138
LEAVE YOUR EGO AT THE DOOR.. 138
STAY CONSISTENT 139
DON'T UNDEREAT 139
STAY HYDRATED 140
PRIORITIZE GETTING QUALITY SLEEP 140
ALWAYS LIFT WITH PROPER FORM... 141
ONLY DO THE RECOMMENDED AMOUNT OF CARDIO..................... 141
STOP MEASURING YOUR SUCCESS AGAINST THE SUCCESS OF OTHERS 142
DON'T BE AFRAID OF SUPPLEMENTS 142

CONCLUSION... 145

REFERENCES 149

Introduction

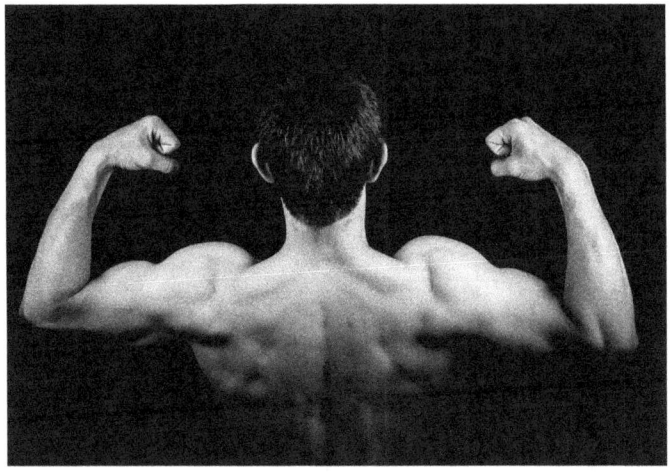

"No man has the right to be an amateur in the matter of physical training. It is a shame for a man to grow old without seeing the beauty and strength of which his body is capable." - Socrates.

Who would have known that one of history's greatest thinkers would have the same kind of passion for physical training that he did for philosophy and contemplation? You can't deny that he has a very strong argument here. As human beings, our very existence is a miracle in itself. Think of how many conceivable determinants needed to be satisfied in order for you to get here - to be who you are right at this very moment. The sheer mathematics of it is almost incomprehensible. It would be an awful waste of your life if you didn't push yourself to find out just how far you can go; to discover how much you can endure; to see how much you can get done.

If you're someone who aspires to have a chiseled and muscular frame, then that's a good thing. There is nothing shallow or pretentious about you wanting to look good and have a better build. Whenever someone tells you that it's really shallow for you to obsess over building your body, just tell them that you have Socrates on your side and that man was far from being shallow. You understand this journey that you wish to embark upon. It's more than just trying to get bigger biceps or a more sculpted chest. It's about what these physical manifestations represent. It's about the hard work and the commitment that you put into getting what you want. By picking up this book, you prove to yourself and the world that you have a curious soul and are eager to learn. You are showing that you aren't afraid of going after what you want. That's always the first step to becoming a better person than you were yesterday.

Of course, having the motivation to do good and make something of yourself is not enough. You also need the know-how and the proper game plan necessary to get you from where you are now to where you want to be. That's precisely what this book is going to help you out with. Whenever you look at the world's elite athletes and see their prime bodies that look like the gods themselves have sculpted them, it can be very easy to become discouraged and think that you would never be able to amount to that. However, you have to understand that all of these elite athletes started out somewhere. In fact, a lot of them may have started out in worse conditions than the current shape that you're in right now. The only thing that separates you from them is the amount of work that they've already put in. Fortunately for you, there is still time left for you to do everything that it takes to get your desired body. This book will help shed light on the art of bodybuilding and all of the science that goes into it. It's imperative that you gain a fundamental academic understanding of how your body works and what you need to do to take care of it. This book will also go into detail into the roles of exercise and nutrition and how you can use these tools to sculpt your dream physical form. Most importantly, this book is going to present to you all of the basic knowledge that you need to design your own path moving forward.

At the end of the day, everyone's bodies are all shaped differently. This is why you must be able to develop a plan for yourself to make sure that it's tailor-fitted to your own personal needs and goals. Don't worry. It's not as complicated as it seems. This book is going to help walk you through the entire process in a very structured and purposeful manner, so you can avoid any misunderstandings about what to do in order for you to achieve your goals.

However, aside from talking about what this book is, it's also important to emphasize what this book isn't going to be. First of all, this book isn't going to do the work for you. Just reading this book alone doesn't guarantee that you're automatically going to get the body that you want. The most crucial step here is for you to apply your knowledge to your everyday life to the best of your ability. This book will not serve as a magic pill that is a one-size-fits-all solution to all of your problems. Understand that all human beings are different. The training plan for an elite athlete is not always going to be effective for a novice or beginner. However, what this book can do is provide you with enough knowledge and perspective to understand the potential and limitations of your own body. It doesn't matter whether you're overweight, differently-abled, or whatever. It doesn't matter if you're allergic to gluten or if you have diabetes. All of the principles that will be presented in this book can still help you out in your fitness journey.

Benefits of Lean and Healthy Muscle Building

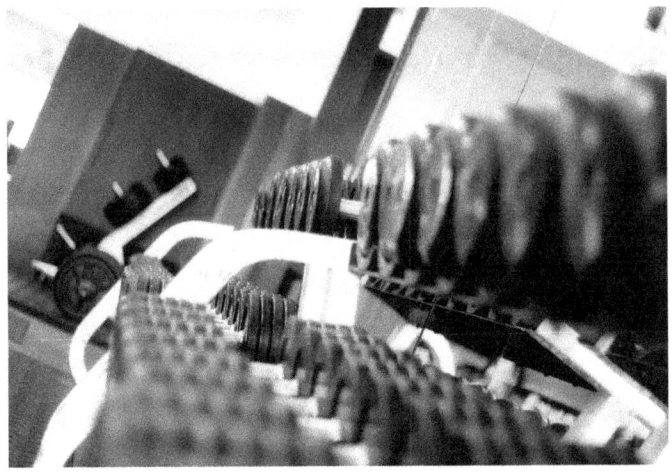

To provide you with more incentive to pursue your goals of getting bigger, better-defined muscles, you should know that the benefits of your hard work exceed mere aesthetics. It's not just about how your body is going to look on the outside. Sure, it can make you feel great to know that you look good. But a lot of the benefits can also be found on the inside. Sure, if you ask many diehard bodybuilders, they will tell you that they derive a lot of joy and fulfillment from being able to achieve their goals. The fulfillment that you get is a benefit in itself, but it's also so much more than that. Sure, weight training is very much concerned with the actual building of a muscle, but there are other physical benefits to strength training as well. This is a common misconception that many have about people who look to build muscle.

Here are just a few of the many ways in which building muscle can lead to you having a better quality of life:

Muscles Help Regulate Blood Sugar Levels

Muscles in themselves don't necessarily regulate the body's blood sugar levels per se. Rather, it's the resistance training that is required for bodybuilding that helps regulate the body's blood sugar levels. In fact, many doctors recommend resistance or anaerobic training for anyone who might have Type 2 Diabetes. This is because strength training helps improve your body's ability to process glucose and deliver it to the muscle, thus decreasing your body's blood sugar levels at any given moment.

Muscles Help Control Body Fat

Muscles are known to help control the body fat levels in your body because they increase your metabolism. Metabolism is essentially the process of converting your body's stored fat into energy for movement and bodily functions. So, the more muscles you have, the more energy that is required for your body to function. The more energy you burn, the more fat that you lose as well. Bulking up isn't just about getting sculpted. It's also about getting rid of that stubborn fat which is proven to be a leading cause for disease in many people.

Muscles Give You More Functional Strength

Getting bigger and stronger as a result of resistance training doesn't just mean that you get to lift heavier weights at the gym. All of this added strength and functionality can apply to your everyday life as well. When you are a stronger person, life just generally becomes easier for you. It won't be a problem having to lift heavy boxes when you move. You won't have to worry about pulling yourself up onto something. The exercises that you do at the gym translate to better efficiency in movement for everyday life. However, this might also mean that your friends will be calling you first when they need help lifting something heavy.

Muscles Reduce the Risk of Cancer and Cardiovascular Disease

Earlier, it was mentioned that muscles help control the level of fat in your body. However, not all fats are created equal. There is such a thing as visceral fat which can be very harmful to your health. Visceral fat is a kind of fat that attaches itself on top of your major organs. All of this added fat can put unnecessary stress on your organs and potentially cause them to malfunction. This means that your major organs like your heart, liver, or kidneys can be compromised and cause some serious illnesses for you. On top of that, visceral fat is also notorious for enabling the development of cancerous tissues. By engaging in regular strength training, you are minimizing the likelihood of developing harmful visceral fat.

Muscles Strengthen Bones, Ligaments, and Joints

Having bigger and stronger muscles will also help make you a more durable person overall. This is especially useful if you're an athlete who always likes to stay active. For example, if you are a long-distance runner, you can still stand to benefit from doing some bodybuilding and strength training every once in a while. Adding more muscle to your frame will help lessen the stress and impact on your joints and bones. Imagine every single step that you take while running and the amount of stress that can have on your knees. If you have stronger leg muscles, they can help take some of the tension away from your joints by absorbing most of the impact.

Muscle-Building Improves Your Emotional and Mental Health

Again, muscles in themselves might not necessarily be primarily responsible for improving your mental and emotional health, but resistance training can help support a healthier state of mind. Whenever you exercise, your brain triggers the release of hormones called endorphins. These are also often referred to as the happy hormones. They are responsible for making you feel like you've accomplished something and they put you in a good mood. They are often described as being able to provide people with a natural high.

Muscles Lengthen Your Lifespan

Lastly, having a lean mean fighting machine as a body is also likely to lengthen your lifespan. For one, we've already talked about how you are less likely to contract certain harmful diseases and illnesses if you have lower body fat and higher muscle mass. That fact alone can really improve your chances of living a longer life. However, having an improved state of mental and emotional health as a result of consistent exercise can also help you live longer. This mental and emotional boost can help you relieve stress, which is known to be one of the biggest killers in the medical world. With consistent exercise, you are also effectively making yourself more invulnerable to stress.

And there you have it. Those are just some of the most important benefits that you can get from devoting more time and effort to sculpting your body. Of course, by now, you're probably raring to go, but you've got to tone it down a little bit. Remember that you need a game plan first. You need to take a structured and methodical approach to develop your physical fitness. The first step to doing so is understanding how your body works and the science that goes into biomechanics, metabolism, catabolism, and other concepts involved in muscle building.

Chapter 1:

An Introduction to Building Muscle

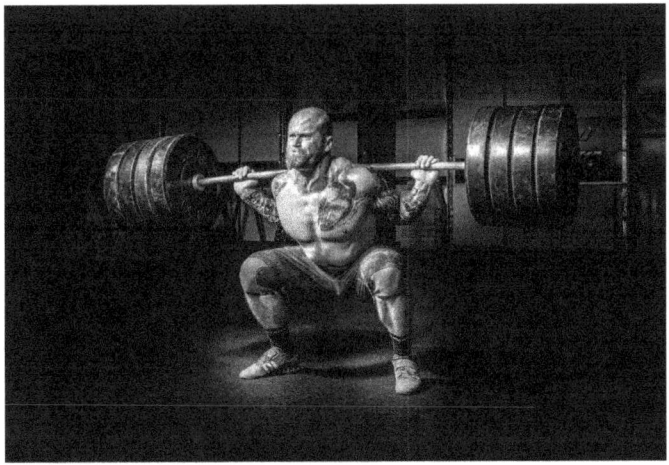

Before we get to the practical aspects of building muscle, we have to discuss the biological first. Don't worry. This isn't going to be some super complex scientific discussion on physiology and biomechanics. You don't need to be a medical doctor or have a specialization in biology for you to understand everything that's going to be discussed here. We are going to keep things as simple as can be. Again, this is a book that is designed for anyone to read and be able to understand. You won't have to worry about encountering ideas or concepts that you wouldn't be able to comprehend or apply to your own life.

In this chapter, we are going to delve deeper into what exactly happens in your body whenever you work out and try to build muscle. Whenever you do a bicep curl, your muscles don't just magically grow ever so slightly with every rep. That's not how the muscle building process works. It's a lot more complex than that. By the time you finish this chapter, you will gain a more profound understanding of how your muscles gain mass and what you can do to stimulate that process.

Consider the knowledge in this introductory chapter as a prerequisite to everything that you'll learn in the rest of the book. This will be the foundation for all of the knowledge that you will absorb and is crucial to your journey towards getting the body of your dreams. This chapter is going to tackle concepts like clean and dirty bulking, hypertrophy, rest and recovery, range of motion, strength imbalance, and more. With this chapter, we are laying the groundwork and the blueprint for the future version of yourself.

How do Muscles Grow? The Science of Hypertrophy

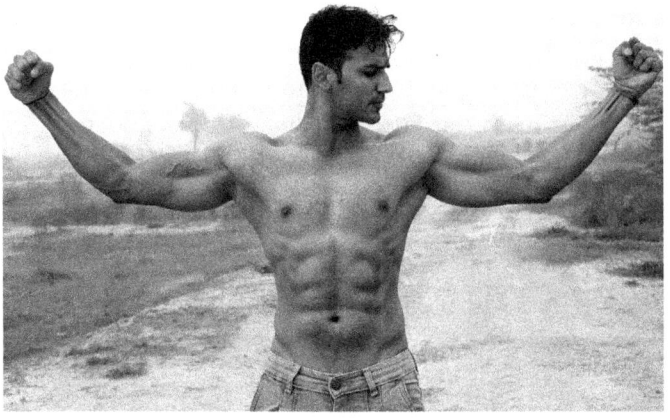

You know that going to the gym, lifting weights, and eating protein can help you bulk up and get bigger. You probably know this because of your exposure to popular media or you might have some friends who are avid gym rats. And yes, these activities can definitely contribute to muscle growth. But how? That's what we're going to try to explain in the simplest terms possible right now. The actual process of building muscle is called hypertrophy. Scientifically, this is the process of the increase and growth of muscle cells in your body. Now, there are two types of hypertrophy that you need to know about, especially when you're planning out your strength and training program. First, there is myofibrillar hypertrophy. This deals with the increase in the size of your body parts that are involved in muscle contraction. Then, there is sarcoplasmic hypertrophy. This is the increase in your muscle's ability to store glycogen. To the layman, these two classifications of hypertrophy might not necessarily be all that important. However, if you're really going to drill down on your training, you need to pay more attention. Myofibrillar hypertrophy has to do with improving your muscle's capacity for strength and speed. This means that your movements are more explosive when you do this kind of muscle building. On the other hand, sarcoplasmic hypertrophy has more to do with sustained efforts and endurance. This kind of training allows you to keep moving over long periods of time.

Now, it still begs the question, how exactly does hypertrophy work? Well, it's all a matter of *breaking to build*. You have to break your muscle fibers down to allow for space for new fibers to grow and add to your mass. It's that simple. Whenever you perform a movement that stresses your muscle fibers at a certain frequency, your muscle fibers will break and become damaged. This is the reason you might feel sore for a day or two after a session of heavy lifting. The soreness that you feel is the damaged muscle fibers in your body. Now, that these fibers are broken, you need to replace them in order to maximize the recovery process by loading up on protein. Proteins are made up of amino acids which play a crucial role in the building of muscle and spearheading the body's recovery. When you consume protein, these molecules enter your bloodstream and travel to the areas of your body where your muscle fibers are broken. Then, they will fill the gaps and add to your body's overall mass.

This might all seem theoretical to you, so let's try to paint a clearer picture of what is taking place in your body when you're trying to build muscle. Imagine yourself performing a few reps of the bench press. This is a movement that requires the effort of your pectoral muscles, triceps, and front shoulders. The more reps that you perform at a challenging weight, the more you are essentially stressing these muscles out to the point of mechanical damage and metabolic fatigue. This means that your muscles are breaking down and are losing the energy that they need to sustain this movement for a longer period of time. This is why the reps on the bench press become increasingly more difficult the more reps you complete.

Over time, as the muscles become bigger and stronger, certain movements become easier to perform. This is why the concept of *progressive overload* is important in building muscle. If we go back to the bench press example, imagine that you start out performing five sets of five reps of the bench press at 135 lbs. three times a week. After the first couple of sessions, it might feel very challenging for you. But then, it gets easier every time. This is because your muscles are growing and learning to adapt to the movement. If you continue to stick to this workout scheme, your muscles will be less likely to break and engage in hypertrophy. This is why it's advisable to increase either the intensity or the volume of your workouts gradually over time. So, after a couple of weeks of lifting 135 lbs with a 5x5 rep scheme, you can try increasing the load or the number of reps. Maybe you can do 145 lbs with the same rep scheme or you can keep the load and add another set to every session. This way, you are constantly stimulating your muscles and challenging them to the point of fibral breakage.

Approaches to Hypertrophy

The Role of Calories in Building Muscle

Now, we've talked about how hypertrophy is essentially a process of breaking to build. You break your muscle fibers down in order to build them up. While there is no other natural way to build muscle other than through hypertrophy, there are still many approaches to the *break to build* method. In particular, there are two main methods that we will be focusing on in this book. There is the slow and lean bulk and the overloaded dirty bulk. Before we can discuss the differences between these two methods of bulking up, you have to orient yourself on the roles that calories play.

When you think of calories in the fitness industry, you might get the impression that these are substances that you need to stay away from because they will make you fat. However, what most people don't realize is that calories in themselves are not fattening. All food contains a certain amount of calories and these calories are made up of vital nutrients that your body needs to sustain itself. Earlier, we discussed how protein is a crucial ingredient to the process of hypertrophy. Every gram of protein that you consume carries around four calories. Without any calories, your body would not be able to sustain itself. You wouldn't be able to survive.

Every single second you're alive, your body is continually using up calories whether you realize it or not. Sure, you might know that performing strenuous movements like running, jumping, and heavy lifting can burn a significant amount of calories. But what you may not know is that you're still burning calories even when you're just lying down. You're even burning calories as you sleep. This is because your calories are converted into glucose which is used as fuel for your body to function properly. Every time your heart beats, it requires energy. Every time your lungs contract and expand, they require energy. Whenever your intestines process and break down your food, they require calories. This means that the food that you eat gets converted into the energy that is responsible for allowing your organs to function properly.

However, calories often get demonized in the fitness industry because many people often overindulge in their food to the point where they are consuming more calories than they are burning up. We all have different caloric requirements depending on how our bodies are made up and the kinds of activities that we do every day. A person with a larger build who works as a hauler for a living will require more daily calories than a slender individual who has a desk job. Now, in terms of training for building muscle, you will require a specific number of calories in order for you to sustain your daily output. If you're not eating enough calories, especially from protein, then you are compromising the entire hypertrophic process. This is because you are not feeding your muscles enough protein to facilitate the building process.

We will go into more detail about calories and general nutrition later on in the book. This is a topic that will require its own chapter and there are many more details that need to be addressed.

Clean Bulk vs Dirty Bulk

When you structure your diet and training scheme, there are two things that you need to familiarize yourself with: caloric deficits and caloric surpluses. You get into a caloric deficit when you consume fewer calories than your body requires to function daily. This can also mean longer recovery times for sore and broken down muscle fibers. You get a caloric surplus when you consume more calories than you are using. This ensures that your body is getting the calories that it needs to function, but if done excessively, it can also lead to weight gain and the development of fatty tissues.

Given that, there are typically two approaches that bodybuilders will take when it comes to building muscle: clean bulking and dirty bulking. A clean bulk is when someone does strenuous strength training and eats just about the right amount of calories that hovers over the line in terms of how much they're burning off every day. So, if you calculate that you're burning off around 3000-3500 calories per day, then that would also be the number of calories you consume when you're on a clean bulk. The pros of this method include you making sure that you are never eating excessively. You are still engaging in hypertrophy while minimizing the development of fat. However, with this kind of dieting method, it's also possible that you aren't eating as much as you should be. Calorie counting is not an exact science. This is why progress might seem very slow and minimal with this kind of approach to hypertrophy.

Then, there is the dirty bulk. This is when you engage in intense strength and resistance training and you eat substantially more calories than you know that you're burning every day. Clean bulking involves you toeing the line of your caloric output every day. Dirty bulking has you going over that line consistently. This might be beneficial to some people who are looking for clearer and more immediate results with their hypertrophy. However, it also leaves most others prone to unnecessary fat gain.

Should You Do Cardio While Building Muscle?

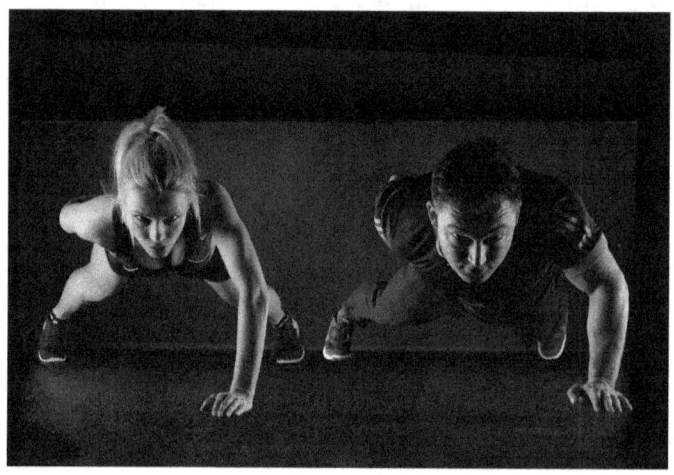

To this day, the fitness community remains divided on the matter and there's a reason for that. There is no direct answer that just applies to everyone. Again, it's always going to be a case by case basis depending on a person's physiological makeup and goals. Don't worry. This is not a cop-out. In general, the answer to "Should you do cardio while building muscle?" is always going to be yes. Cardiovascular exercises are good for the heart and they can benefit everyone. However, that isn't the right question to ask. Rather, the right question lies in *how much* cardio should you be doing when you're trying to build muscle. But in order to answer that question, there are two other questions that you need to address first.

What is your body type and what are your goals?

Addressing Your Body Type

Are you a naturally skinny person who seems to always stay lean no matter how much you eat? Do you already have a big build but it's made up mostly of flab? Are you the kind of person who seems to gain muscle relatively easily? These are all questions that you need to ask yourself in order to determine your body type. We will delve deeper into the science of body types in the next chapter. But for now, what you need to know is that the more fat you already have in your body, then the more cardio that you need to do. Of course, building muscle through strength and resistance training can also help facilitate fat loss. However, you can supplement your fat loss efforts by doing more cardiovascular activities like running or jumping ropes.

Catering to Your Goals

Another important detail that you need to take into consideration is what goals you have for yourself. As a general rule of thumb, the leaner and more defined you want your muscles to appear, you might have to do a little more cardio than the typical bodybuilder. However, if you're someone who is focusing more on bulk and you don't care so much about definition, then you shouldn't really concern yourself too much with cardio at all.

Bottom Line

This is why the fitness community continues to be so divided when trying to answer this question. No one answer is suitable for all bodybuilders. It's all subject to your own personal interpretation of your situation and your goals. Ultimately, the best that you can do is analyze the most ideal theoretical framework to follow and adopt it for yourself. If you get the results that you want, then that's great. If you don't feel like you're progressing over time, then don't be afraid to go back to the drawing board.

The Importance of Sleep and Recovery

We won't delve too much into this concept for this initial chapter because it's far too complex and it requires a full chapter on its own. However, it's still essential to stress the importance of incorporating sleep and recovery into planning for your muscle building process. There are plenty of people who will come up with the most detailed diet plans and the most comprehensive training programs for you to follow and that's a good thing. But it's also important that you develop a good sleep and recovery plan for yourself as well. Good sleep is what enables you to have the energy every day to sustain your strenuous workouts. Your recovery time is also important as this is where the "build" aspect of the *break to build* process takes place.

The time you spend at the gym training is you breaking your muscles. The time you spend recovering is your body building itself up. Again, this is something that you will be briefed on more comprehensively in a later chapter. But for now, it's important that you know that sleep and recovery are integral aspects of the muscle building process.

Chapter 2:

Understanding Your Body Type

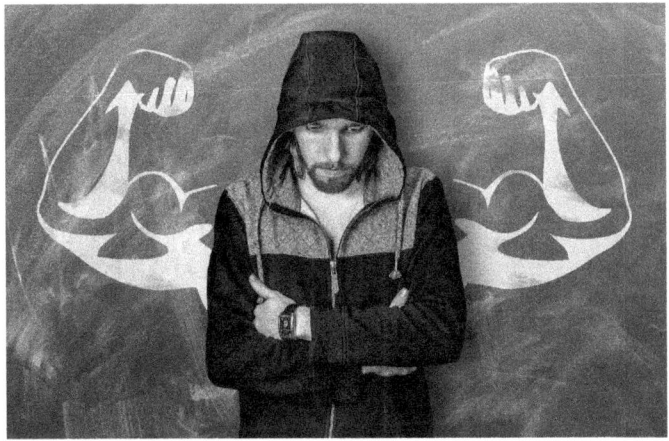

Not everyone is going to be wired the same way. This is why the concept of bodybuilding is a lot more complex than most people make it out to be. A training program that proves effective for one person isn't necessarily going to be one that works for another. You and a friend might share the same personal trainer and the same training routine, but you might not necessarily get the same results. You might be doing all of the same things, but your bodies might be responding differently.

This chapter will give you more insight into the different body types and how they are different.

It's important that you really understand your body type because it is the most important tool for achieving optimal fitness. The most important tool is not a barbell. It's not a dumbbell. It's not a squat rack. It's your body. This is why you need to take some time to really understand your body's ins and outs to determine your body type. Once you are familiar with your body type, then you will be in a better position to plot your point of attack for your fitness goals and objectives.

The Three Main Body Types

There are three distinct body types that most people typically tend to fall under, in bodybuilding. These body types can have a dramatic impact on how your body responds to training stimuli, nutrition, recovery, and other factors that are involved in building muscle. Given that, gaining knowledge of the ins and outs of your body type will allow you to understand what you need to do in order for you to find success. It was mentioned that there are three distinct body types that we will be discussing here, however, it's important to note that you're not necessarily just bound to one category all of the time. Sometimes, people can start out as one type when they are younger and then gradually transition to another body type as they get older. There are a variety of factors that go into determining your body type, such as genetics, lifestyle, physical activity, health history, and more. With that reminder out of the way, let's get right into discussing the differences between being an ectomorph, endomorph, and mesomorph.

Ectomorph

The first body type to be discussed here is the ectomorph. This is the type of person who struggles to gain weight despite feeling full whenever they eat. The ectomorph struggles to gain fat or muscle and is often referred to as *hard gainers*. When trying to build muscles, ectomorphs will have to consume a lot more lean protein (sometimes, with the help of supplements) in order to see results. Also, ectomorphs tend to progress more slowly when it comes to building strength as compared to the other body types. Whenever they don't eat enough, they are also prone to losing weight a lot more quickly than others.

The main reason that ectomorphs struggle with weight gain is because of their fast metabolism. They have bodies that are so efficient at processing carbohydrates and converting them into fuel for energy that none of these get left behind in the body as stored fats. As much as possible, ectomorphs need to limit cardiovascular activity so as not to lose any unnecessary calories that might compromise the muscle building process.

What Does an Ectomorph Look Like?

Typically, an ectomorph who doesn't work out or doesn't do any kind of resistance training will have the build of the stereotypical marathon runner. They might have visible abs as the result of not having any fat around the belly rather than from core exercises. Sometimes, ectomorphs can still have a little fat around the body, but the fat will still be contained in a relatively small frame.

The Dos and Don'ts of an Ectomorph

The first thing that you need to remember as an ectomorph is that you need to stay away from the treadmill as much as possible. There's no need for you to be doing cardio. In a bodybuilding program, cardio is typically used as a tool for burning fat in order to highlight the definitions of muscles. However, since you're an ectomorph, your body is already doing a good enough job of burning fat on its own. If you do cardio, you risk burning more calories than you would typically want and your muscles end up getting broken down and converted into energy as compensation.

Ideally, you will want to perform compound movements for a huge bulk of your training regimen. These are movements designed to recruit different muscle groups to accurately and safely perform a given task. Also, look for high volumes in terms of rep schemes. This is the best way for you to progressively build your strength given your body type.

Lastly, you want to make sure that you have a high-calorie diet. Again, your body type is one that enables the fast processing of food and the burning of calories. This means you have to constantly replenish your energy stores so that your body doesn't end up breaking your muscles. Go for a lot of healthy complex carbs and lean protein to help you bulk up. Healthy fat from olive oil or nuts is also good for helping your body process nutrients more efficiently. Fats also carry more calories per gram relative to the two other macronutrients. Also, don't be afraid to make use of supplements to make sure that you are getting all of the nutrients that you need to sustain your workouts.

Endomorph

An endomorph is someone who is very good at retaining fuel storage. They tend to have higher amounts of fat and muscles concentrated on the lower extremities of the body. Many trainers and experts will say that endomorphs have the most difficult time in terms of managing weight and developing overall fitness. If you are an endomorph, gaining weight is going to be a relatively easy process for you. Conversely, losing weight and cutting fat is going to be more difficult for you than it is for others. You will have a tendency to have a wider torso and legs. It's very easy for you to build muscle, but it's hard for you to gain LEAN muscle. That means that while you may be building your muscles through caloric surpluses, it's also likely that you're getting fatter at the same time.

Of course, this isn't to say that getting a lean and trim body is totally impossible for you. There are many endomorphs out there who have chiseled physiques as the result of their hard work and strict commitment to their fitness regimens. You just have to make sure that you really put in the hard work at the gym and in the kitchen with your diet. Getting strong is very easy for you, but losing the fat while maintaining that strength might prove to be a challenge.

What Does an Endomorph Look Like?

If you are an endomorph, it's likely that you will have what most people refer to as a stocky or blocky build. You might have a wider rib cage than most and your hips might be just as wide, if not wider than your collarbones. You might also have thicker joints and flabbier limbs than most. Muscle definition is still possible in endomorphs, but they are likely to be accompanied by lumps of fat as well. The most prominent endomorphs in the sporting world tend to be American football players, sumo wrestlers, and Olympic weightlifters.

The Dos and Don'ts of an Endomorph

The first thing you could be doing wrong as an endomorph is spending hours at a time on a treadmill or elliptical machine. Sure, it might seem like a good idea to devote more time to cardio work since you aren't necessarily built lean, but, this wouldn't be an efficient use of your time, especially if you're looking to build muscle. Rather than doing slow steady-state cardiovascular work, try using bursts or intervals of high-intensity training instead. You get all of the benefits of the fat burn while you're exercising, and you get to rev up your metabolism for when you're at rest as well. For example, instead of running at a steady pace on a treadmill for 30 minutes, try doing a 15-minute interval of 30-second sprints and 30-second walks.

Another thing that you should do is lift heavier loads. You might believe that, since you're on the stockier side, you need to focus on shedding fat before building muscle. However, you can use muscle building as a tool for you to burn fat more effectively. The best way to do this is to lift heavy weights at low to moderate reps with minimal recovery periods in between sets.

In terms of your diet, limit your carbohydrate intake as much as possible. This will force your body to turn to your stored fats as a source of fuel. Also, load up on a lot of lean protein and fiber. This is just to make sure that while your body is burning stored fat for fuel, your muscles are constantly being fed. This means you need to stay away from food like bread and rice. Focus more on green vegetables as a source of carbohydrates.

Mesomorph

When it comes to body types for bodybuilding, you must consider yourself blessed if you are a mesomorph. You have the type of body that is most primed for building lean muscle without gaining too much fat. It's relatively easier for you to get that athletic build that you want than it would be for an endomorph who leans towards being stocky and an ectomorph who is skinny. There are plenty of people around the world who look like they are athletes despite having poor nutrition and exercise regimens. These are the ones who are likely to be considered as mesomorphs.

However, it's important to remember that body types aren't always set in stone. Just because you might be a mesomorph in your teens and early twenties doesn't mean that you're going to stay that way. A lot of the time, as you get older, your metabolism slows down and it'll be harder for you to keep the fat away. This is why it's still important for mesomorphs to incorporate healthy training and nutrition habits into their daily lives if they are to remain healthy and fit. Being a mesomorph puts you at a physiological advantage when competing against the other two body types. But that doesn't mean that you shouldn't be putting in the time and hard work necessary for you to get the real body you want.

What Does a Mesomorph Look Like?

Ultimately, a mesomorph is someone who looks like they spend a considerable amount of time at the gym even when that isn't the case. Also, mesomorphs are those who tend to pack on muscle relatively quickly. They also find it a lot easier to gain strength and explosiveness in a relatively short amount of time. Like an endomorph, you are likely to have wide shoulders and a strong-looking chest. However, you're going to be a lot trimmer around the waste as compared to the endomorph. You are less likely to develop belly fat.

You are also more inclined to develop sculpted legs, particularly with the quadriceps and calves.

The Dos and Don'ts of a Mesomorph

Again, since mesomorphs are typically blessed with good genetics, there is a high chance that they will become complacent with their diet and training. This might not necessarily be a problem at the start. However, over a sustained period of time, this can prove to be very harmful. This is why mesomorphs need to establish more measurable and tangible goals for themselves. This way, they stay more motivated to workout as they chase real targets.

Also, incorporate regular progression in your workouts as much as possible. Again, you are blessed with good genes and you will likely develop your strength at a far more rapid rate than the other two body types. This means that you need to constantly be upping your workout's difficulty so that your progress never stagnates. If you make your workouts difficult, this means that you are bringing new stimuli every single time you train. Also, try to incorporate more explosive movements into your training routine. Focus on functional movements like box jumps, sprints, pull-ups, and other training tools that translate to function in everyday life.

Final Thoughts

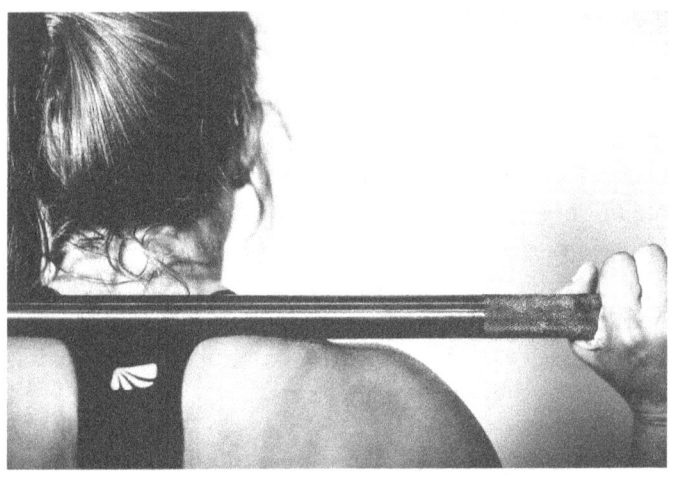

Regardless of whatever body type you fall under, there's no need to feel discouraged because of the genetic makeup of your body. Sure, you might feel like other people will have an advantage because they have a certain body type. But the struggle is all the same. At the end of the day, no one gets their ideal body without putting in the hard work. It doesn't matter whether you're an ectomorph, endomorph, or mesomorph. If you're lazy and unmotivated, you aren't going to get results. Ultimately, it helps to have better tools that will help you to succeed. However, all of these tools are pointless unless you put them to good use.

Having an ideal body type is an advantage. But not having an ideal body type should not be a deterrent either. Keep in mind that the journey that you're about to embark on is yours and yours alone. If other people are progressing faster than you, it's irrelevant. You are the only person that you need to be focusing on here. Just because you know that your body type has certain advantages or disadvantages relative to other people is not the point. The point of this entire chapter is to point out to you how your body responds to certain stimuli so that you can design the most ideal training plan that caters to your specific needs.

It can be so easy to look at your body and become discouraged because you might not necessarily have the natural body type you want. However, that is not a viable excuse for you to avoid putting in the work. In fact, gaining more knowledge about your body type should serve as an incentive for you to try even harder. The smarter you are about the physiological makeup of your body, then the better position you will be in to find success in getting the body that you want.

Chapter 3:

Nutrition

Contrary to popular belief, building the perfect body isn't just about what you do in the gym. You can do all of the bicep curls and back squats in the world. But if you have terrible eating habits, you're never really going to maximize your body's potential fully. You can't outrun a bad diet, both literally and figuratively. It's that simple. This is why this portion of the book is going to focus more on the work that you do in the kitchen as opposed to the gym. You will come to realize that everything that goes into your mouth can do a lot more for your body than anything that you can do with a barbell or weights.

You will find that this is a pretty consistent theme in this book, but there isn't really any one way to go about dieting. Different diets can have different effects on different people. You've already gotten a glimpse of that earlier when we talked about the different body types and how these people carry different needs both in training and in nutrition. This chapter isn't necessarily going to advocate for one particular diet over another. Don't expect that. Rather, what you can expect is to gain a more in-depth understanding of fundamental nutrition principles so that you can figure out what kind of diet would suit your body type and training regimen best.

In this chapter, we're going to touch on the basics of macronutrients and why you need to be paying attention to them. We are also going to take a deeper dive into the concept of metabolism and calories, and how you can construct your own metabolic plan based on your lifestyle and body type. You will also be briefed on some examples of healthy food items and meals that you should be incorporating into your diet. Finally, you will be given some concrete tips and tricks that will help you make the most of your diet as you pursue your goal body.

The Role of Nutrition in Building Muscle

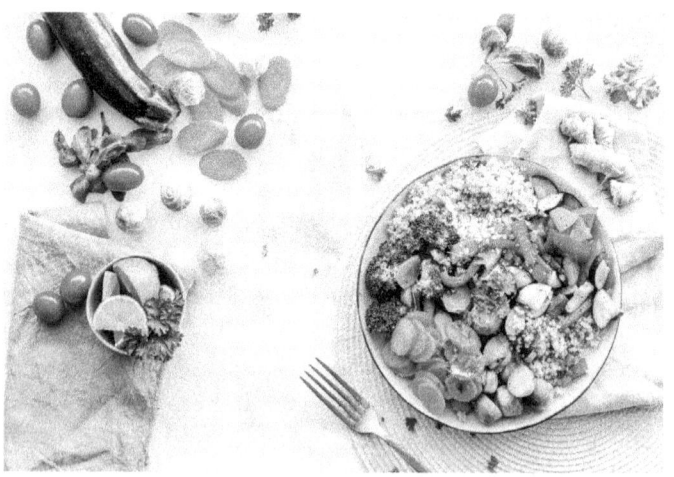

It's time for a hot take: you're wasting your time at the gym if you're just going to eat a lot of crappy food for every meal. You probably already know from your lessons as a kid that you need to have a well-balanced diet in order for you to stay healthy. This is why, as a child, you were always force-fed vegetables even though all you probably wanted to eat were hotdogs and cereal. Hopefully, you've outgrown that phase and have developed a more sophisticated palate. Of course, there are still some adults who might be eating more vegetables now than they did back when they were younger. But how much is the appropriate amount? Should you be eating more meat? Isn't eating meat supposedly bad for you? Are all fats bad? Then why do some people say that there's such a thing as good fats?

These are all very valid questions that you might have. Nutrition is a messy game and this is why a lot of people become intimidated before starting a new diet. However, the more that you study nutrition and its basic principles, the simpler and clearer everything becomes. This is especially true if you're the kind of person who pays a great deal of attention to how your body looks and how it functions. And if you're reading this book, then there's a good chance that you are indeed that kind of person.

Building the optimal body is not a feat that can be achieved by hard training alone. Again, this is a break-to-build process and the training that you do in the gym is merely the breaking aspect of it. The food that you put into your mouth is responsible for building your physique. For one, food is going to help give you the strength and energy to complete your workouts. Also, food is responsible for strengthening your muscles and joints to the point where they increase your build and overall physique.

That is exactly how you should view your relationship with food. You would never be able to perform well at the gym if you're not eating right. Also, you wouldn't be able to grow your muscles if you aren't feeding them properly. The role of nutrition in building muscle is two-fold. It impacts both your performance and your body's overall aesthetics. If you obsess over the amount of weight that you pull and the number of reps that you execute, then you need to do the same with your food as well. You have to obsess over the number of calories that you eat and how much protein you're taking in. These are all little details that can add up over time to a dramatic impact and success for your body.

The Value of Protein

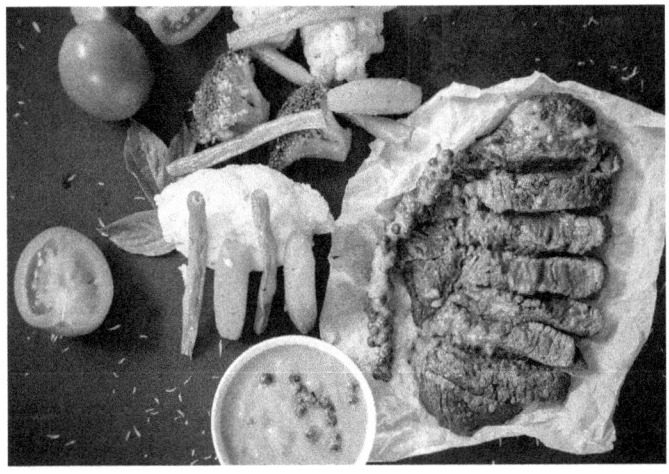

You probably already know by now that bodybuilders and athletes live off protein. But what you may not know if you're a nutrition novice is that protein only comprises one of the three macronutrients that you need to be incorporating into your diet. Yes, protein serves as a very important building block for feeding your muscles and strengthening your joints. However, you can't just live off protein alone. You need to understand the relationship that protein has your body and the other macronutrients as well. This way, you have a more holistic approach to understanding your nutrition and developing a plan for yourself.

Figuring Out the Three Macronutrients

If you recall all the old lessons you had about nutrition, you might remember that every food item might be rich in a particular nutrient. Also, you might recall that every nutrient carries a distinct benefit for your body. For example, you might have been told that carrots were rich in Vitamin A. This meant that you would have improved eyesight. Also, you might have learned that oranges are rich in Vitamin C. This means that they can help you improve your immune system. Now, it's good if you really familiarize yourself with all these nutrients and what food you can source them from. However, for the purposes of building muscle, there are only three nutrients that you *need* to really pay attention to. They're referred to as the *macronutrients* and they comprise carbohydrates, fat, and protein.

In this segment on nutrition, you are going to be briefed on the different values of each macronutrient and what roles they play in your quest to build your physique. Again, it's not just about eating as much protein as you can. You don't want to be a meathead. Once you have a better understanding of all three macronutrients, you will be in a better position to have a truly more well-balanced diet… the same one that your grade school teachers and parents tried to teach you about when you were younger.

Carbohydrates

The first macronutrient that you need to know about is carbohydrates or carbs for short. Too often, carbs will get a bad rap in the fitness community because they are closely associated with food like donuts or pizza. Naturally, if you are eating a diet that consists of copious amounts of those particular food items, you're going to get fat. However, while these high-carb food items might be bad for you, carbs in themselves aren't so bad.

In terms of calories, carbs only carry four calories per gram. This is substantially much fewer calories per gram than fat. However, the problem with carbohydrates when it comes to building muscle isn't just about how many calories they have. It more has to do with how your body is processing those calories internally. Carbs serve as readily available sources of fuel for your body. If your body detects carbs in your system, it immediately begins processing those carbs to be converted to glucose. This glucose is what will serve as fuel for you to run, jump, lift, breathe, and anything that requires the recruitment of any part of your body. So, if you're someone who trains in the gym regularly, then you need your carbohydrates to fuel your workouts. Sometimes, you might even get that little extra push during your training sessions as a result of carb consumption. Although, any leftover carbs that aren't processed for energy will be turned into stored fat for future use. It's essentially your body's way of preparing itself in case you need a quick supply of energy in the future but don't have any immediate access to food.

Given that, it's important that you only consume as many carbs as you need at any given time. This way, you are assured that you are only using up the exact amount of carbs that your body needs to sustain movement and none of it will get turned into stored fat. Now, the exact amount is going to differ from person to person depending on training intensity, volume, and body type. However, a general rule of thumb is that the number of carbs you should be eating should be around twice the number of grams of protein that you're consuming. If you're an endomorph who gains weight quickly, you might want to be more conservative with this approach and lower the number of carbs to maybe around 1x-1.5x your protein consumption.

Now, the conversation with carbs doesn't stop there. You also have to know that there are two different types of carbohydrates: *simple* and *complex*. The simple carbs work as fast-acting sources. They're the carbs that you need to get the job done quickly and efficiently. They're readily available and they run out just as fast. Then, there are the complex carbs. It takes longer to process the complex carbs, but they offer a more sustained steady stream of energy to the body. Think of simple carbs as energy for workouts like short sprints while complex carbs are more beneficial for marathons. Later, we'll go into detail about certain examples for both kinds of carbs.

Fat

The next item on the agenda is fat. Contrary to popular belief, eating fats don't necessarily make you fat. Again, like carbs, fat has gotten a very bad rap in the fitness community because of its name and the number of calories that it carries per gram. For one, some people think that the fat that they have around their bellies, arms, or thighs is the result of the fat that they consume from oil or meat. But that's not necessarily how fat works and that's not how your body processes fat either. Just because you eat the fatty part of a steak doesn't mean that it's going to translate into fat on your belly.

Fat is a very powerful micronutrient that helps your body absorb and process all the other essential nutrients that it needs to function properly. So, in a way, they are crucial to the muscle building process as they help your muscles absorb more protein and recover from strenuous workouts more efficiently. Fat is also responsible for improving your body's immune system and they can also be tapped as a potential energy source for whenever your body runs out of carbohydrates.

Like carbs, not all *fatty* food items are created equal. Fat can be categorized into two distinct types: *saturated* and *unsaturated*. Essentially, you can tell the two apart based on how they appear at room temperature. Typically, unsaturated fats take on a liquid form at room temperature while saturated fats retain their solid form. When incorporating fats into your diet, you want to make sure that you're sticking to unsaturated fats as much as possible. These are the types of fat that are responsible for providing all the positive health effects on your body's internal processes. Conversely, diets that are rich in saturated fats are often associated with diseases like stroke, cardiac disease, and hypertension.

Protein

Lastly, there is protein - every bodybuilder's favorite macro. Proteins consist of different types of amino acids. They are often referred to as the building blocks of any muscle tissue. Think of a big strong house and picture its sturdy walls and protective roof. That house wouldn't be as strong and sturdy as it is without the cement blocks that were used to fortify that structure. Protein essentially serves as the cement blocks for your body. This is why protein is immensely popular in fitness, especially for building strength and muscle.

Now, what are some of the practical benefits of protein exactly? Well, first it's about increasing strength and mass. The more protein that gets fed into your muscles, the stronger and bigger they're bound to become. This is why it's completely pointless for you to be lifting a bunch of weight at the gym but not eating the proper amount of protein to supplement it. All of your efforts will end up being wasted. Also, protein is in charge of facilitating your body's recovery process after going through vigorous workouts. It can help repair any breaks that take place in your muscle tissues and joints to make sure that you come back stronger and fitter than before you started working out. Protein is also low in calories as compared to fats. Like carbs, a single gram of protein only carries four calories. However, it's important that you still do not consume more protein than is required. If you're eating a lot of protein, but aren't doing the resistance training that necessitates a high consumption, then all of that protein will be turned into fat. You have to do strength training to create those breakages in your muscle fibers where protein can swim to and repair. If these breaks don't exist, then the protein you eat will be processed and turned into stored fat instead.

Of Calories and Metabolism

We've already touched on these two concepts in the first chapter of this book. Now, we're going to shift things up by taking a more practical and applicable approach to the ideas in this segment. Before we do that, let's go through a brief refresher. Any food that you eat carries a certain caloric value. For example, a medium-sized egg can have as much as 70 calories and a cup of rice can have around 250 calories. The reason that foods have calories is that they are made of nutrients that feed and nourish your body. The calories in your food are processed by your body and then utilized as fuel for daily function. If you eat calories in excess of any energy you're expending, then you're putting yourself in a caloric surplus. If you're not eating enough calories, then you're going into what is called a caloric deficit.

Now, how do you know how many calories you're burning in your body? That all depends on something called metabolism. This is your body's ability to take the calories you consume and convert it into energy. The higher your body's metabolism, then the more calories that you burn at any given moment. The converse is true should you have a slower level of metabolism. Given that, if you have a higher metabolism, then you would burn more daily calories than someone else with lower metabolism even though you eat the same amount of food. If you have more calories left over in your body, then you are likely to gain weight over time. If you eat fewer calories than you're using up, then you will end up losing weight.

But how do calories affect your weight gain exactly? Well, to put it to a numerical value, a single pound of fat equals around 3,500 calories. So, if over a week your total caloric deficit amounts to 3,500 calories, then you will be one pound lighter than the week prior. If you flip it and have a 3,500-calorie surplus, then you will gain a pound of fat over a week instead. When it comes to muscles, it's a little more complicated. A single pound of muscle is only composed of 700 calories. However, that doesn't mean that eating 700 calories will lead to you gaining a pound of muscle. It's estimated that you need to consume around 2700 - 3000 calories from lean protein in order to gain a pound of muscle.

Figuring Out Your Base Metabolic Rate

Now, you might be feeling a little overwhelmed right now with all of the nutrition knowledge that's been discussed so far. Don't worry. Ultimately, the only thing that you need to know about calories and metabolism is that it's a game of pluses and minuses. The more calories you have at the end of the day, the more pounds you will gain and vice-versa. Also, the higher your body's metabolism, then the more calories you will be able to burn in a day. Great. So, now that's out of the way, you need to get to work on figuring out just how many calories you're using up in a day. Sure, there are smartwatches and fitness trackers out there that may give you a rough estimate of how many calories you're using up daily. But it also pays to be able to make these computations on your own. Not everyone is going to want to shell out cash for these fitness trackers that aren't guaranteed to provide data that is 100% accurate anyway.

Before we can get to discussing the *hows* of computing for your base metabolic rate, we have to make sure that you understand what a base metabolic rate is and *why* it's important, to begin with.

The thing about your body's metabolism is that it's always at work even when you don't realize it. You might just be sitting in front of your computer or lying down in bed. Your body is still trying to convert calories into energy. Basic bodily processes like breathing, cell regeneration, blood circulation, and digestion all require energy. Most people might jump on a treadmill and see that they're burning a certain number of calories during a single running session. But the calories you burn during exercise aren't the only calories that you burn throughout the day. Your body also burns calories at other points during the day in order to sustain itself. The rate of your calorie-burn outside of exercise is referred to as your base metabolic rate.

Now, it's important for you to figure out your base metabolic rate so that you know how many calories you should be consuming in order to sustain yourself without getting fat or losing muscle. Again, if you eat too much, you might end up gaining weight. If you eat too little, your body won't recover as quickly from training sessions and you will struggle to gain lean muscle. Computing for your base metabolic rate or BMR is as simple as following this no-fuss formula:

For Women:

BMR = 655 + (9.6 × weight in kg) + (1.8 × height in cm) − (4.7 × age in years)

For Men:

BMR = 66 + (13.7 × weight [kg]) + (5 × height [cm]) − (6.8 × age [years])

What would this computation look like? Let's say you're a 29-year-old man who stands 180 cm tall and weighs 85 kg. To compute for your BMR, it's merely a matter of substituting values.

BMR = 66 + (13.7 x 85) + (5 x 180) - (6.8 x 29)

= 66+ (1164.5) + (900) - (197.2)

= 1,933.3

So, based on these computations in this example, you would be burning 1,933 calories daily outside of any additional calories burned from exercise. Again, BMR doesn't take into consideration any amount of training that you might be doing. If you really want to dial in on how many calories you're burning daily, then you have to first assess how active you are. Try to fit yourself into one of the following categories:

1. Sedentary - minimal to no exercise (multiply BMR by 1.2)
2. Lightly active - light exercise 1-3 times a week (multiply BMR by 1.375)
3. Moderately active - moderate exercise 3-5 times a week (multiply BMR by 1.55)
4. Very active - hard exercise 6-7 times a week (multiply BMR by 1.725)
5. Extra active - very hard exercise 6-7 times a week (or if your profession is physical in nature like construction work, athlete, etc.) (multiply BMR by 1.9)

Of course, these are just rough estimates. It's not an exact science. The numbers might be skewed depending on a variety of factors. Take whatever results you get from these computations as ballpark figures that you should be aiming for and adjust your training/diet plan accordingly. If you see that the results are good, then stick with it. If you feel like your computations are off, then make the necessary adjustments.

Caloric Surplus or Deficit?

You might already have a fairly good understanding of how many calories you're burning each day based on your body type, age, gender, and level of physical activity. You were able to compute your base metabolic rate and you also multiplied that amount based on how much physical activity you engage in over a week. Now, it's time for you to try to figure out how much you should be feeding yourself. Depending on your relationship with food, you may or may not like what you're about to read here. For some people, eating large amounts of food (especially bland healthy food like greens and chicken breast) can be a struggle. For many, cutting out bad food like sweets and junk food can be an even bigger tragedy. However, no one ever said that getting the body of your dreams was going to be easy.

In this segment, we are going to delve deeper into the idea of caloric surpluses and caloric deficits. What are the benefits of either and when are they useful? Ultimately, it's as simple as determining what your goals are. If you are an ectomorph or a mesomorph with a relatively skinny frame, then you should look into having a caloric surplus. Your body is burning so much fuel and energy to compensate for your level of physical activity. If you want to build lean muscle, then it's important that you feed your body adequately with healthy lean proteins and complex carbs. You don't want to be going into a caloric deficit because this will hinder the process of hypertrophy in your body. However, your approaches to caloric surpluses should be different. If you're an ectomorph, you have a little more wiggle room and a higher margin for error with regard to how many excess calories you can consume daily without getting fat. If you're a mesomorph, you want to be very careful to not overdo it with your caloric surplus. A general rule of thumb is to not exceed an excess of 500 calories per day so that you maximize muscle growth and minimize fat gain.

If you're an endomorph, then your margin for error is a lot slimmer as compared to a mesomorph and ectomorph with regard to staving off fat. It's so easy for you to gain weight even when you're training really hard at the gym. While it's okay in some instances for you to go into a caloric surplus, it's not an absolute necessity. Sometimes, you would be better off at just balancing out your calories burned and calories consumed entirely. In some cases, endomorphs can still even gain muscle while going into a caloric deficit so long as they are getting most of their calories from protein. However, if you really want to go into a caloric surplus, make sure that you don't exceed 300 excess calories daily and incorporate more cardio into your training.

Structuring Your Diet Plan around the Three Macros

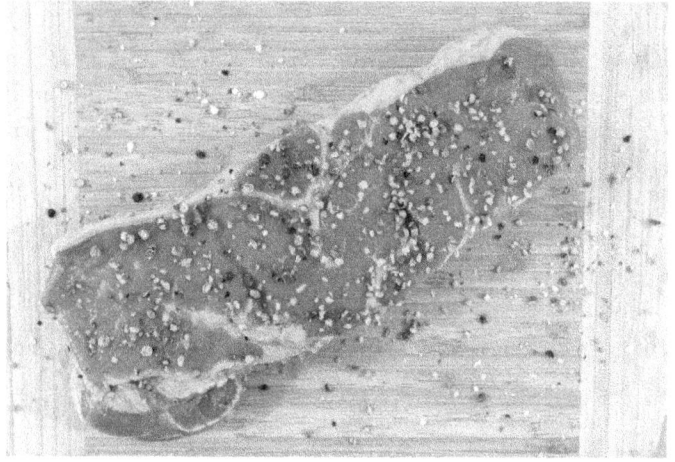

You might be growing a little frustrated over how theoretical a lot of these concepts have been so far. You already know about calories burned and calories consumed. You're already familiar with surpluses and deficits. But how is that knowledge going to translate to the amount of food that you should be eating? In order for you to create an effective diet plan for yourself, then you need to utilize your knowledge of the three macronutrients.

What Should Your Plate Look Like?

It would be ideal if you pay close attention to every single nutrient that goes into your body. However, it's also quite impractical. You don't always have to stay on top of how much sodium, potassium, or vitamin C that you're getting with every meal. The more practical way of paying attention to your nutrition is by looking at your macronutrients. There are some people who want to take a more detailed approach to dieting where they really count the numeric values for calories and macronutrients. This is a great way to really drill into the dieting process, but it isn't necessary. Sure, there are a lot of fitness and dieting apps along the way that can help you track what you're eating and how much of it translates to certain nutritional values. However, all that really matters is that you eat enough that makes you feel like you can sustain your physical performance and functionality every day.

If you want to take a more hands-on approach to tracking your food, then go ahead. Make use of a traditional food journal or embrace technology and use apps like MyFitnessPal to help you document your food more intensively. But for a lot of people, a simple eye test would suffice. If you're interested in building lean muscle while staving off fat, try to maintain a 40-30-30 ratio for calories that you consume in a day. What this means is that of the total amount of calories that you eat daily, 40% should be made up of protein sources, while 30% should come from each of the other two macros, fats, and carbs. To illustrate this further in numbers, imagine that you have a prescribed diet plan of 2500 daily calories in order for you to have a healthy caloric surplus.

40% of 2500 = 1000 calories

30% of 2500 = 750 calories

Given that, you should aim for a macro distribution of 1000 calories worth of protein, 750 calories worth of fats, and another 750 calories from carbs.

However, these values are not absolute. Again, there are plenty of variables that come into play here. Mostly, the ideal distribution of macros here all depends on your goals. If you're looking to trim down, it might be best for you to opt for a higher protein count. So, maybe you can go for a 50-25-25 or 50-30-20 breakdown. It all depends on how your body will respond to certain dietary formats. You have the freedom and wiggle room to play around here to see what works for you.

Keep in mind that as you progress in your bodybuilding journey, your body is going to respond to food intake differently over time. A lot of the time, you will find that you will hit certain plateaus in your fitness journey. If this is the case, the first thing that you have to do is adjust your training. Take note of the principle of progressive overload. You need to be making your workouts more and more challenging as you get stronger. If that still doesn't work, then you might have to tweak your diet. If you're not progressing as quickly as before with regards to building muscle, then you might have to up your calorie or protein intake. Perhaps you're getting a little pudgy and gaining a little bit of unwanted fat. This might be a sign for you to lower your calorie intake and carbohydrate consumption.

Best Food for Carbohydrates

Ideally, carbs should cover around 30% of your total caloric intake every day. However, not all carbs are created equal. You want to make sure that you are sourcing your carbs from whole foods that add more nutritional value to your diet plan. 300 calories from steel-cut oats are not the same as 300 calories from ice cream. One contains a lot of healthy fiber that will help your digestive system while the other is loaded with unnecessary sugar that will give you insulin spikes. Whole foods tend to also make you feel fuller for longer. This means that you won't have those random cravings in the middle of the day for unhealthy junk. Here are a few examples of the best food sources for carbohydrates:

- steel-cut oats
- whole wheat bread
- brown or red rice
- whole wheat pasta
- green leafy vegetables (lettuce, cabbage, spinach, kale, etc.)
- tomatoes
- bell peppers
- quinoa
- sweet potatoes

Best Food for Fat

For the most part, you just want to stay away from food items that have a high amount of trans fats in them. They are referred to as bad fats because they are notorious for negatively impacting a person's cardiac health and overall immune system. Instead, shoot for generous amounts of unsaturated fats and moderate amounts of saturated fats. These are fats that carry a lot of antioxidants and natural nutrients that will help regulate your body's internal processes.

Unsaturated Fats

- olive oil
- nuts
- nut butters
- peanuts
- seeds (pumpkin, sesame, etc.)
- fatty fish (salmon, mackerel, etc.)
- vegetable oils (canola, corn, sunflower, etc.)
- avocadoes

Saturated Fats

- cheese
- butter
- cream
- fat from meat
- coconut oil
- palm oil

Best Food for Protein

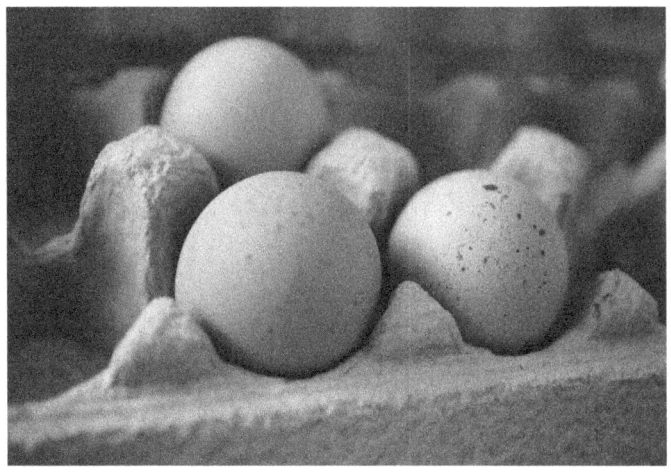

Lastly, of course, there is protein. You already know that protein serves as the cement blocks that will build the foundation of your body's musculature. So, in any type of bodybuilding-focused diet, you want to make sure that you are getting a generous dose of healthy lean protein from natural food sources. Most of the time, you can get protein from meats like beef, chicken, pork, and fish. However, it's also possible to get protein if you're on a plant-based diet. Here are some of the most common sources of protein from food:

- eggs
- milk
- cheese
- chicken
- pork
- turkey
- beef

- fish
- nuts
- beans
- legumes
- yogurt, etc.

Top Foods to AVOID at All Costs

Discipline is a very important trait to master when you're trying to build your optimal physique. A lot of people tend to get hung up on the aspect of discipline that focuses on establishing new routines and adopting new habits. However, not a lot of people realize that discipline also has to do with getting rid of bad habits that might be detrimental to you pursuing your goals. There might be certain food items in your current diet plan that you need to eliminate altogether if you really want to maximize your strength and resistance training endeavors. Here are some common culprits of food items that might keep you from achieving your goals:

Alcoholic Beverages

As painful as it might be, you're going to have to part ways with your favorite beers, whiskeys, tequilas, and vodka cocktails for a while. The sad truth is that alcoholic beverages can inhibit your body's ability to process the nutrients that it needs to sustain itself. This means that the muscles that you break from resistance training aren't going to be repaired as efficiently with protein when you have alcohol running through your bloodstream.

On top of that, you are taking on a lot of unnecessary calories when you go out on a night of binge drinking with friends. A single serving of beer can often contain as much as 150 or even 200 calories. You might opt for harder liquors that have relatively lower calorie counts, but if you mix them in with other ingredients like sweeteners or sodas, then it's all moot. An occasional beer every now and then isn't going to be so bad for your body. Just try to make sure that you limit the alcohol intake as much as possible. If you can, try eliminating it from your diet altogether.

Refined or Added Sugars

In general, food that is high in refined or added sugars add very little value to your body's nutritional intake. Of course, it can be very tempting to reward yourself with a delicious donut or a pint of ice cream after a hard workout. However, you would also be effectively undoing a lot of the progress that you make in the gym. Instead of getting leaner and gaining more muscle, you are only adding sugars to your body which will get converted into stored body fat and cause you to crash and burn. Instead of rewarding yourself with sweet treats after a workout, opt for healthier options like a fruit smoothie or some low-carb protein bars.

At the end of the day, there's no denying that a good old chocolate bar is going to taste much better than a bowl of kale. But no one ever said that dieting was going to be easy. Try to limit your consumption of food items like sodas, sugary sports drinks, sugary coffee beverages, ice cream, cake, donuts, cookies, potato chips, and the like. They're okay for occasional treats, but you shouldn't be making it a habit of consuming these items consistently.

Deep-Fried Food Items

Just because chicken is filled with a lot of protein doesn't mean that you should be eating buckets of fried chicken for every meal. Working hard at the gym doesn't give you an excuse to line up at KFC every day. The truth is that these deep-fried food items like fried chicken and french fries are laden with a lot of unnecessary calories that come from fat sources like oil and carb sources like breading and flour. On top of that, these deep-fried items can promote inflammation in your body and can slow down the muscle recovery process.

Common examples of deep-fried food items are fish fingers, chicken nuggets, fried chicken, potato chips, french fries, onion rings, corn dogs, and more.

Best Supplements for Bodybuilders

Now, it's time to discuss the idea of supplementation. The first thing that you have to know about supplementation is that it isn't necessarily a requirement in order for you to build lean muscle. If you really commit to having a clean and healthy diet, then you are going to find success in your goals in fitness. However, for a lot of people, one can only get so far on food alone. There are just some people who will find it difficult to stuff themselves with pounds of lean chicken breast every day in order to meet protein requirements. This is exactly where supplementation comes in.

There are a lot of people who might be hesitant to try supplementation at first because of a certain reputation that these substances might carry. There are many novices who might lump healthy and natural supplements along with performance-enhancing drugs like steroids. These are not the same. It's important to emphasize that it's perfectly safe to make use of health supplements in proper moderation. Your relationship with supplements should be the same one that you have with your food. You should only be taking in what your body needs to perform optimally. Also, supplements should be seen as something that *accompanies* a proper diet based on food. They shouldn't be acting as meal replacements. As much as possible, you want to source your nutrients from whole foods that are as natural as can be.

Having said that, you can still benefit from cycling supplements into your daily dietary rotation. You just have to know what specific supplements to look out for, how much of them you need, and what purposes they might serve in your training regimen. In terms of bodybuilding, here are some of the top supplements that you might want to invest in.

Whey Protein

The first supplement that you want to invest in is whey protein. This is essentially one of the most popular supplements out there for bodybuilders. This is because of the fundamental bodybuilding aspects that protein has on the body. Ideally, whey protein is a product that is consumed immediately after a hard workout. Preferably, within 30 minutes. This is because whey is a fast-acting protein and is absorbed by the muscles quickly. A lot of modern whey protein manufacturers also market products in a variety of flavors. Whey protein usually comes in a powder form and can be mixed in with other ingredients like milk, juices, or blended fruits. This can make whey protein a perfect go-to treat or reward after a difficult workout.

Casein Protein

Casein protein is another kind of protein supplement that usually comes in a powder form as well. However, it differs from whey protein in terms of the time that it takes to be processed. Whey protein needs to be absorbed into the body within 30 minutes after a hard workout in order for one to yield optimal benefits. This is because whey mostly acts within a short amount of time. With casein, it's different. It's a much slower process. Most people drink casein protein before going to sleep. This is so that your body is receiving a constant flow of protein all throughout the night. Studies have also shown that the muscle recovery process heightens during the sleep stage.

Weight Gainers

If you are someone who gains weight easily like an endomorph or a mesomorph, then you might not want to invest in this product. However, if you are an ectomorph who struggles to pack on the calories that are required to build muscle, then you can try out weight gainers. Usually, these are powdered substances that are loaded up with a lot of protein, either whey or casein. However, aside from that, they are also loaded with carbohydrates to add to the calories per serving. Again, make sure that this supplement is only used alongside a healthy diet plan that revolves around real food. It shouldn't serve as a meal replacement.

BCAA (Branched Chain Amino Acids)

Typically, branched-chain amino acids or BCAA consist of three essential acids that are crucial for building muscle: leucine, isoleucine, and valine. Typically, you would be able to source these acids in incremental amounts through meats, poultry, dairy, and fish. This is essentially a supplement that is meant for people who don't eat enough protein from whole foods in their diet. Again, not everyone is going to be happy with stuffing themselves with chunks of chicken breast or tuna for every meal. This is where supplements like BCAA come in to help you get the nutrients that you need without having to eat an uncomfortable amount of food.

Creatine

Aside from whey protein, there are plenty of bodybuilders who will say that creatine is their go-to supplement. First of all, creatine is responsible for taking all of the water that you drink and feeding it into your muscles. Almost 80% of your muscles are made up of water and creatine helps make sure that your muscles always stay hydrated. Aside from that, it is also responsible for providing energy to your muscles so that they are always optimized for peak physical performance whenever you're working out. It's a lot easier to build strength and mass through a regular intake of creatine. However, there are detractors who will say that creatine can damage your kidneys or liver because it takes all of the water you drink away from these organs and feeds it into your muscles instead. This is why it's important that you stay hydrated and drink a lot of water whenever you are on a creatine cycle.

Omega-3 Fatty Acids

You might be familiar with Omega-3 Fatty Acids as those nutrients that are always found in fish oil gels. This is a supplement that is particularly popular among the elderly as it is often marketed as a product that helps with joint pains and aches. However, more than just strengthening your joints, fish oil can also help the recovery process by decreasing the inflammation in your muscles. This means that you will tend to feel less sore after a hard workout and it will be easier for you to exert more effort in the gym the next day.

Caffeine

Yes, caffeine. Not a lot of people may realize that caffeine is a very popular dietary supplement for athletes and people who stay active in general. Caffeine is especially popular among bodybuilders for two reasons. One, it increases the body's metabolism. This means that it helps the body burn more fat while at rest. The other reason that caffeine is so popular is that it provides athletes with the energy and stamina that they need to sustain difficult workouts. Marathoners and endurance athletes are popularly known to take caffeine prior to a race. However, bodybuilders also usually take caffeine prior to a heavy lifting session in order to provide more energy to the muscles.

The Best Nutrition Secrets, Tips, and Tricks

Nutrition is a complicated topic. It's possible that you're feeling a little overwhelmed with everything that has been discussed so far, and that's okay. This is not something you should expect to master in a day. These are all very complex ideas that you need to gradually integrate into your daily life. It's not something that you can just fully absorb in one go and then be done with. Given that, perhaps it's best to summarize all of the knowledge into bite-sized tips and tricks that you can apply to your everyday life.

Again, your success is ultimately going to be determined by the habits that you practice every day. If you just try to apply these simple secrets and tips to your life on a consistent basis, you are bound to see results. And you won't even have to wait too long to feel like you're progressing.

Prioritize Real Food

Again, it's important that you prioritize real food. And when we say *real food*, we mean food that undergoes the least amount of processing as possible. Avoid overly processed goods such as canned meats, bagged chips, chocolate bars, and the like. These are not *real food* and they aren't going to help you get the body that you want. As much as possible, try to focus on sourcing your meals from meats and plants. Try to keep it as clean as possible.

Don't Be Afraid of Supplements

Now that you know that you have to prioritize real food always, let's talk about the value of supplements. Ultimately, you want to prioritize real food as much as you can. However, there will be times where you just can't get the nutrients that you need from whole foods alone. This is where supplementation can really help you out. For instance, you might be reaching your caloric limit for the day, but you still need some extra protein. A nice glass of whey protein can help you meet your protein needs without you having to find a chicken to munch on at the end of the day or after a workout.

Drink Lots of Water

Again, water is life. Literally. You have to make sure that you stay hydrated whenever you're looking to build muscle. For one, your muscles are made out of water. In fact, your entire body is made out of water. You want to make sure that your body is hydrated so that it would be able to function properly. Also, staying hydrated helps your cells regenerate faster and it can aid in muscle recovery as well. It can also be very dangerous to your kidneys if you are consuming a lot of protein without drinking an ample amount of water. Eating too much protein and not enough water can compromise the integrity of your kidneys.

Track Your Food Intake

You definitely want to keep track of the food that you're eating. There is no way that you would be able to maximize your potential and achieve the goals that you want just by winging it. Sure, there are some people who are experienced enough to know how much they should be eating without keeping a food journal. However, this only comes through consistent practice and experience. If you're a novice and you're just starting out, you really need to take the time to track what you're eating as accurately as possible. This might seem like it's a lot of work to do, but no one ever said that this was going to be easy.

Plan Your Meals

Tracking your meals might seem like such a hassle. However, if you engage in meal planning and preparation, then everything becomes a lot easier and simpler. All it takes is just one day of a week for you to sit down and write all the meals that you'll be eating over the course of seven days. Write everything down and include all the major meals along with your snacks. This is beneficial for numerous reasons. For one, it makes the grocery shopping process a lot simpler. You will only end up buying the ingredients that you need for your meal plan. Next, it will be easier for you to track your meals and caloric intake when you've planned them out beforehand. It's also going to help keep you from overeating or undereating throughout the week whenever you have a plan to follow.

Make Adjustments Whenever Necessary

The diet plan that you start with isn't necessarily going to be the diet plan that you stick with for the rest of your life. You have to understand that your body is going to go through some significant changes as you get older and fitter. This is why it isn't always going to respond to a particular diet plan the same way forever. It's important that you continually reassess the effectiveness of your diet plan. If you notice that you aren't getting the proper results, then be open to tweaking your diet a little bit to accommodate for the changes in your body or workout routine.

When Unsure, Eat Meat and Vegetables

There will be times where you won't be able to figure out what you should be eating. This is especially true whenever you find yourself having nights out with friends or family at restaurants. You might be forced to stray away from your meal plan and order something on the spot. Don't worry. Just remember that you can never go wrong with lean meats and vegetables. When in doubt, order a salad and a meat of some kind. Make sure that there is a minimal amount of sauce and dressing. This way, you know you are still eating clean even when you're eating outside.

Fibrous Carbs Over Sugar

Carbs are not the enemy here. Hopefully, you will have learned that when you were reading about the macros and the different roles that they play in building muscle and staying healthy. You should always look to incorporate carbs into your diet to a certain extent. However, whenever you do eat carbs, always try to prioritize fibrous carbs over sugary ones. Go for carbs like wheat and grains because they help aid in your digestion and body's processing of nutrients. Sugar is just going to give you unsustainable energy and unwanted body fat.

Avoid Alcohol

Just avoid alcohol. Avoid drinking beers and wines because they're loaded with a lot of calories and carbohydrates. Also, avoid drinking cocktails because they usually have a lot of unwanted carbs and sugars in them as well. Hard liquors might seem okay because they are low in calories, but they can really compromise your body's ability to absorb protein. So, just try to avoid alcohol to the best of your abilities. Of course, this doesn't mean that you can't have alcohol for as long as you live. Which brings us to our next and final tip...

Treat Yourself (Sometimes)

Have an occasional cheat day. Go ahead. Life isn't worth living if you're not having fun. At the end of the day, you really need to learn to enjoy the process if you're going to find success in it. There's nothing enjoyable about being strict and always disciplining yourself. Sure, you're going to find a lot of success that way. However, you should never pursue success at the cost of your own happiness. This is why it's good if you have an occasional cheat day. Even as a reward system, this can be a very good practice to have in your fitness journey. For example, you can reward yourself with a scoop of ice cream after a week's worth of strict dieting. Maybe you can go out on a one-night drinking binge after gaining 5 lbs. of muscle to celebrate. Just make sure that these treats are done very rarely. They might not be good for your body, but they're good for your soul.

Final Thoughts

By now, you should be convinced that diets are very important in determining how your body is going to respond to training stimuli. You are never going to progress as quickly or as efficiently as you should be in the gym if you're not supplementing your workouts with proper nutrition habits. As tempting as it might be to just indulge in a diet of pasta, pizza, burgers, donuts, cookies, ice cream, and beer all of the time, you're going to have to develop your sense of discipline. To reiterate a point that was made at the start of this chapter, you can't outrun a bad diet. If you're continually eating junk, then your body is never going to achieve everything that it's designed to achieve.

It can be so easy to fall into the trap of thinking that just because you're working hard at the gym, this means that you can eat whatever you want. This is absolutely the wrong mindset to have when it comes to designing your diet plan. True fitness is a healthy collaboration of both physical training and nutrition. You need to marry these to concepts in order for you to achieve optimal health and wellness. A failure to conflate a good training regimen with proper diets can result in suboptimal results. It's just that simple.

Hopefully, this chapter will have given you good insight and sufficient motivation to pursue a healthier lifestyle in the realms of the kitchen. Not all battles take place on the race track or in the boxing ring. Master the art of proper dieting and nutrition to win the ultimate war against unwanted body fat.

Chapter 4:

Rest and Recovery

It's not always just about working hard. Fitness and nutrition aren't only about the work you put in the gym or your dieting discipline. It's also about how you take care of your body in terms of rest and recovery. Sure, it can get pretty addicting to just spend all day every day at the gym when you're just starting out. This is especially true if you've managed to find a lot of success instantly. That success can become addicting to the point where you crave it over and over again like a drug. So, since you've found success by working hard at the gym, you think that you can get more of it by spending time at the gym. In theory, this can be true. However, in all practicality, you're only human and you need to rest. In fact, you might be doing more harm than good to your body if you don't give it the proper care that it needs in order for you to carry on towards achieving your fitness goals.

This chapter is going to turn the spotlight towards the importance of recovery, sleep, and just taking care of your body in general. Whenever you start working out, it can be pretty amazing to witness all of the remarkable things your body can do. You would never be able to imagine yourself lifting certain weights or defining particular muscle groups until you see them happening. There are some people who go their whole lives thinking that they could never deadlift twice their bodyweight. And it's only because they never think to even try it. So, when you see that your body is performing these amazing feats, it can be tempting to just keep on pushing. However, the problem with that is that you end up putting yourself in danger of injury whenever you don't allow yourself the chance to rest or recover.

There are many ways to approach keeping your body safe and primed for action in the gym every day. A lot of it has to do with certain exercises or habits that you can employ, such as mandatory rest days and supplementation. Sleep is also an important factor that you need to take into consideration here. Try working out while running on less than four hours of sleep and compare it to when you work out after feeling fully rested. You will inevitably find a significant difference in how you feel.

Aside from allowing yourself a chance to recover, there is also the matter of making sure that you keep yourself safe from injuries through *prehab*. Remember that in medicine, prevention is always better than the cure. Don't wait for yourself to get injured or become overworked before you start doing soft tissue work or stretching. These are all concepts that are going to be discussed in greater detail all throughout this chapter. Again, it's not just about going hard at the gym and being disciplined in the kitchen all the time. This is the other less exciting, less glamorous, and more boring aspect of fitness. However, there is no denying just how important these lessons are.

The Importance of Rest and Recovery

All of the successful people you will ever meet in your life will tell you that their success is built by hard work. No exceptions. You can never achieve your grandest goals and dreams unless you put forth the willingness to work hard and suffer for them. It can be so easy to get lost in the romanticism of pouring your blood, sweat, and tears into achieving what you want. This is a concept that is often sensationalized in contemporary media. But do you know the part that rarely gets advertised? Rest and recovery. Picture a superhero movie. You are always so used to seeing Captain America and the Avengers in action fighting against the evilest villains in the world. You see them fight and claw their way to victory. It's very exciting. But what don't you see? You never see Captain America taking a nap. You don't see Batman taking the time to do mobility work for his muscles. You will never see Superman say that he needs a rest day.

Wake up. You're not a superhero and you don't live in fantasy land. You might feel like your body is capable of a lot, and that's a good thing. It always pays to be confident. However, you have to make sure that you don't overstretch yourself here. You are capable of great things, that's true. However, you also need to rest and recover from greatness every once in a while.

When you go to the gym, you are expected to give it your best every single time. And as you engage in hard training, your muscles will break themselves down further and further. You've already learned about this in previous chapters. You know that breaking your muscles down is an important step in the process of hypertrophy. As you break your muscles down, you inevitably become weaker in the short-term only to come out stronger in the long-term. However, getting long-term muscle gains is not achieved merely through hard work at the gym or through proper dieting. There is another dimension to that: rest.

Again, you get weaker in the short-term after a tough training session. Rest and recovery are responsible for making sure that you come out stronger than ever before. When you take the time to rest, you are giving your muscles a chance to heal from being broken down and beaten up. Once you recover through resting, your muscles will feel refreshed and equipped to move heavier loads at more rapid paces. You also already know that hard training can lead to a number of physiological benefits for the human body. Improved blood flow, heart health, respiratory function, digestion, and others are among the benefits you stand to gain from exercising regularly. However, if you don't allow an ample recovery period for your body in between training sessions, these benefits become compromised. Besides that, engaging in what is referred to as *overtraining* can lead to experiencing performance plateaus and injuries.

What is Overtraining?

One general principle that you can apply to any aspect of life is that anything done in excess is bad - even things that you might think are good for you. This, of course, includes training and exercise. Now, it can be very difficult to define what overtraining is because it's a sensation that can vary from person to person. A professional runner might be capable of covering 100 miles per week, while the average joe would only be capable of 20 within the same span. Anything beyond that would be *overtraining* for Joe and just another regular work week for the professional. It's all relative. In this segment of the book, you will be given insights into how you can personally assess whether you are overtraining or not.

There are many factors that can influence a person's capacity for training. Of course, a lot of it has to do with that person's training experience or current level of physical fitness. However, there are also more nuanced factors such as genetics, age, muscle composition, diet, and whatnot. A general rule of thumb is that an average of around 48 to 72 hours of recovery is required in between intense strength training sessions. However, this length of recovery can lessen for those who can gradually increase their workload capacity.

Signs of Overtraining

Now, how would you be able to tell if you are overtraining? It would be nice if you got yourself a licensed professional to oversee your training so that you wouldn't have to worry about details like these. However, if you don't have the luxury of getting personalized instruction from a professional, then you might need to do these assessments on your own. Fortunately for you, it's not that complicated of a process. At the end of the day, the best person to determine whether your body is overly stressed or not is yourself. There are a few signs or *symptoms* of overtraining that you can be on the lookout for whenever you feel like you're overdoing it at the gym. These signs can be divided into physical and emotional/behavioral classifications.

Physical

- persistent muscle soreness
- joint pain
- fever
- elevated blood pressure
- elevated heart rate
- decreased appetite
- unintended weight loss

Emotional/Behavioral

- irritability
- insomnia
- depression
- anxiety
- lack of motivation

The Importance of Sleep

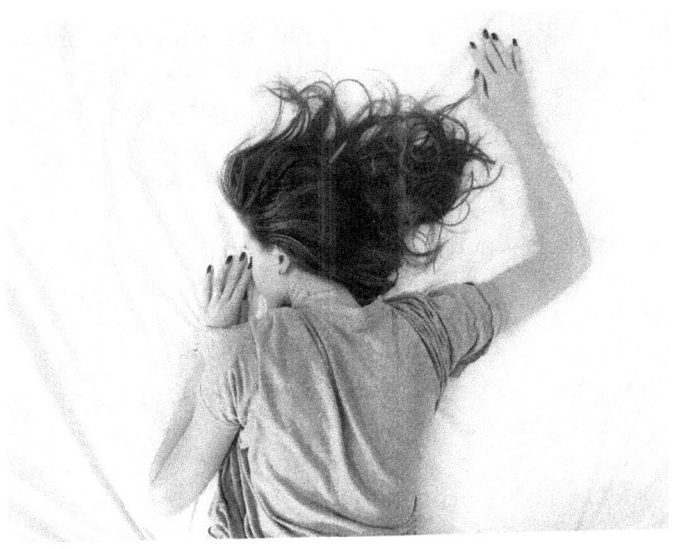

Many working adults will know that sleep is a very precious resource that not many people will have the luxury of getting enough of. Too many times, people will take not just the quantity of their sleep, but also the quality of their sleep for granted in favor of productivity throughout the day. However, while it might make more sense to stay up a couple of extra hours at night to get more things done, it can actually be counterintuitive to your desires to be more productive. In fact, compelling evidence suggests that going multiple days in a row without getting adequate sleep can lead to you feeling groggy and fatigued throughout the day. Therefore, it will be much harder for you to stay focused and motivated to accomplish specific tasks.

It's the same with bodybuilding as well. You might not think much of the amount of time that you devote to sleep. However, you may not realize that the quantity (and quality) of your sleep can have a significant impact on two things: the way that your muscles repair, recover, and grow along with the way that you perform while you're training. Essentially, the time you sleep is when your body goes into a deep hibernation and self-repair mode. Your mind shuts itself down and focuses on repairing the body and preparing it for another day of the usual activities. You're doing so much more than just resting your eyes and brain while going to sleep. You are rejuvenating your entire body. If you compromise your sleep, then your muscles won't end up getting as much recovery as they should. In the end, they won't repair and grow as efficiently as you may have initially wished.

As a byproduct of not allowing your body to recover properly due to a lack of sleep, you can expect suboptimal output and performance whenever you put your body to work. Your muscles never got the chance to repair and rejuvenate themselves properly. So, you might end up still feeling sore and tired when you go to the gym. As a result, you wouldn't be able to maximize your workout because of how fatigued you feel. It's important that you really understand why sleep is important and how you should be integrating proper sleeping habits into your routine.

Understanding the Sleep Cycles

It's been mentioned a couple of times that it's not just the quantity of sleep that you need to be paying attention to. It's just as important that you take note of the quality of your sleep. And before you can really understand what that means, you have to learn about the various sleep cycles.

When you go to sleep at night, there are various stages that you go through. It's a cycle; a repetitive process that has you going from being awake to being immersed in a truly deep sleep over and over again until you wake up. Most people can go through three to five cycles of sleep per night, but it varies from person to person.

Stage 1: Awake

This is usually the stage where you're still slightly awake but you're gradually drifting off to sleep. You might have experienced this when you catch yourself dozing off in the middle of watching TV or while reading a book. During this stage, your senses start to lull themselves and your heart rate begins to slow down.

You're not entirely asleep, but you're not fully awake either. This is the transitory period of you shifting from a conscious state to an unconscious one.

Stage 2: Light Sleep

The second stage of sleep sees your brain and muscles winding themselves down. Your brain activity decreases significantly and your muscles will relax to the point where they lie in a completely static state. Usually, you enter the light sleep stage around 15 to 30 minutes after falling asleep. This is the stage of sleep where you are most easily awakened either by outside noise or physical prompts. Hence, it's called the light sleep stage.

Stage 3: Deep Sleep

The deep sleep stage is the one you want to get the most out of when you talk about bodybuilding and muscle recovery. Deep sleep is the quality sleep that you always want to aim for when it comes to repairing your body. This is the stage of sleep where your brain and muscle activity really goes down to the point where the activity is practically nonexistent. Your heart rate is also probably at its lowest possible point during this time. Usually, people enter a deep sleep stage within 45 minutes to an hour of falling asleep. If you get woken up from a deep sleep, you will feel very groggy and disoriented. You wouldn't automatically be able to discern your environment and it will take a while for your mind to orient itself with what's going on.

Stage 4: REM or Rapid Eye Movement

Try observing your pets whenever they go to sleep, especially your dogs. You might see that they're moving their eyes around rapidly even though they're closed. This is a sign that they've fallen into the REM stage of sleep. This is typically the age of sleep where your brain starts becoming active again and triggers your eyes to move around involuntarily. This is also the stage of sleep when your dreams take place. Most people's nightly sleeping time is around 25% of REM sleep. During this stage, your muscles will become paralyzed and your heart rate will gradually rise.

Negative Effects of Sleep Deprivation

Sleep deprivation is one thing that you always want to avoid when you're trying to live a healthier and fitter lifestyle. Whenever you don't get enough sleep at night, you will feel the negative effects almost instantly the moment you wake up. Depriving yourself of sleep every once in a while is one thing. However, if you do it consistently, then you're going to feel the significant weight of these negative effects more immensely. It's not just about feeling sleepy or tired all throughout the day. There are other physical, mental, and emotional effects that take place whenever you lack sleep as well.

As a bodybuilder, you already know that lacking sleep can slow down the muscle building and recovery process. On top of that, it can also lead to poorer neurological fitness. This means that neurological aspects of fitness like balance, accuracy, timing, and coordination are likely to be compromised whenever you lack sleep. In addition, sleep deprivation also promotes inflammation in the body. This means that swollen muscles will stay swollen for longer and will make you feel more sore than necessary.

Other negative effects that are associated with sleep deprivation include unintended weight fluctuations, mood swings, sugar cravings, lack of focus, and a weaker immune system. Working out while being deprived of sleep can also leave you being more prone to injuries.

The Importance of "Pre"hab

This entire chapter has been dedicated to principles that are focused on taking care of your body as you continually put it through various stress-inducing environments and conditions. That's exactly how you should see working out and dieting. They are stressful conditions that you put your body through in order to harden it and induce self-development. However, it's not good to just always be exposing yourself to such stressful conditions without taking the time to just take care of yourself as well. Remember that the goal here is to participate in the whole marathon. It's not an all-out sprint right out of the gate. You need to make sure that you are playing the long game.

Your days don't always have to be spent lifting heavy weights. You want to work hard, but you shouldn't be working yourself to muscle failure every single time.

This would be the quickest way to get yourself to a physical therapist's clinic for treatment. When building the body of your dreams, the last thing that you would want is to get sidelined for a prolonged period because of an injury. It's not just about safely executing the movements at the gym. It has more to do with what you're doing outside of your regular working sets.

This segment of the chapter is going to delve deeper into the idea of mobility and active recovery days. Just because you want to build muscle doesn't mean your exercise routine should be totally composed of resistance training exercises. Yes, recovery through sleep is important, but that's not the only thing that you can do to make sure that your body is always primed and ready for a hard workout.

Understanding Mobility as a Tool for Injury Prevention

You probably aren't going to get as many likes on Instagram if you post a video of yourself foam rolling instead of you lifting heavy weights. Mobility will never be as flashy or as exciting as actual strength and resistance training, but that shouldn't take away from its importance. Mobility is a very important aspect of fitness that you should incorporate into your routine even though it's not something that everyone likes to talk about. Now, what is mobility exactly? A lot of people seem to confuse mobility with flexibility even when the two are different. Flexibility is the ability of your muscle to stretch or elongate to a certain length. On the other hand, mobility is your body's ability to maintain strength and control while expanding your range of motion. Anyone who is flexible enough can touch their toes without bending their knees. But a person who is mobile would be able to get into a deep squat without having their muscles collapse or give in.

Now, why is mobility important for you as a bodybuilder? It all has to do with you maintaining strength and control as you engage in various explosive movements that are involved with resistance training. There are some people who might be able to bench press their bodyweight. But if you ask these same people to squat with their hip creases getting below the knee, they will cry out in pain. This might prevent that person from getting the potential strength gains that one might earn from engaging in the full range of motion for a movement. If you're doing just a half squat because your lack of mobility prevents you from going the full range of motion, then you are effectively limiting the potency of the movement. You aren't engaging as many muscle groups as you should and your strength gains will be impacted. So, that's one aspect of how mobility can be beneficial for you as a bodybuilder.

Another reason why mobility is important is that it will save you from potential injuries. Too often, athletes who lack proper mobility and who push themselves in training will end up getting tears in their muscles or ligaments. This is because they push their bodies beyond their capacity and the stimuli become too much for the body to handle. There's a reason why immobile people feel pain whenever they are made to squat or fully extend a press overhead. There's something wrong that's going on with their joints and fascia that is preventing them from doing the movement pain-free. Whether as a result of adrenaline or sheer will, some athletes would be able to push past that pain and execute these movements despite their lack of mobility. That pain is supposed to serve as a safeguard or a limiter. But once an athlete continuously pushes past that pain, the body just gives up.

There are various ways in which you might choose to go about improving your mobility. One common method of building mobility is doing light range-of-motion exercises or dynamic stretches. These are different from static stretches where someone holds a stretch for a prolonged period of time. These range-of-motion exercises or dynamic stretches are more kinetic in nature and they require constant movement. They are designed to activate muscles and loosen up tight spots, especially those that are found near joints. Another way of improving mobility is by doing soft tissue work whether through foam rolling or by using a lacrosse ball. Think of your muscles as something that is made up of tiny little threads called muscle fibers. Whenever you do resistance training, these threads become stressed and they can sometimes get entangled. These entangled threads can lead to you experiencing discomfort or having a limited range of motion when you exercise. You can make use of tools like foam rollers, massage guns, or lacrosse balls to help loosen and untangle these muscle fibers so that you regain full range of motion again. You may also use the services of a licensed massage therapist who can work on these problem areas on your body for you.

Active Recovery Days

Being a bodybuilder doesn't mean that you should just be doing bodybuilding exercises every day. Your body needs a break from that particular stimulus in order for it to recover and come back stronger. There are even some people who stick to a training regimen for too long to the point that their bodies acclimate to that routine. When that happens, they experience a plateau in their progress because their bodies aren't responding to the training stimuli in the same manner as before. This is why it's important for you to break your routine up by incorporating occasional rest days or cross-training. If you feel like you have too much energy to go a full day without doing any kind of exercise, then you can have an active recovery day.

Of course, the first option would be for you to just have an all-out rest day. Take one day away from the gym and don't do any exercise at all. During rest days, it's important that you still stay strict on your diet, especially when you're trying to lose fat by going into a caloric deficit. Remember that you're not burning as many calories during these days because you're not going to the gym.

Another option that you can take is by doing an active recovery day. This means that you take the time to do some form of exercise that is less intense and has a different stimulus as your regular routine. This could be anything from shooting hoops in your backyard or doing a quick yoga session. You can even just take some time to do some foam rolling and myofascial release on yourself to work on your mobility. The idea here is that you are still doing some form of exercise without stressing your body out too much, the same way that you would on regular training days.

Best Sleep and Recovery Habits

Track Your Sleep

Again, it's not just a matter of merely getting your *eight hours* every night. You should also be paying attention to the quality of your sleep. This is why it might be wise for you to invest in a sleep tracker. Most modern fitness tracking devices these days have a built-in heart rate sensor that can help track your sleep cycles at night. These devices will tell you how much time you're spending in each stage of a sleep cycle and how many cycles you go through every time you fall asleep. Tracking your sleep for the long-term will also give you a better picture of how your performance might be given certain sleeping patterns. Your data might tell you that you perform better during the day (and during training) when you get x amount of sleep a night.

Stay Away from Blue-Light Devices Late at Night

Unfortunately, we are surrounded by devices that emit blue light every single day. Your television screens, computer monitors, and smartphones all emit blue light. This blue light isn't just straining your eyes, they're also keeping you from falling asleep. This blue light sends certain signals to your brain that mimic the rays of the sun. So, your brain ends up getting tricked into thinking that it's still daytime even when you're supposed to be falling asleep already.

Don't Drink Coffee Beyond 2 PM

Caffeine is a stimulant that increases your heart rate and gives you energy. Having an increased heart rate and restless energy are two things that will keep you from falling asleep. Therefore, it should be common sense that you avoid taking any sort of caffeine too close to bedtime. The duration of the effects of caffeine can vary from person to person, but a general rule of thumb to follow is that you should never drink coffee beyond 2 pm, especially if you're looking to be in bed by nine or ten at night.

Avoid Taking Long Naps During the Day

Power naps are great so long as they are executed properly. When you are sleep deprived, it can really help to just take a few minutes during the middle of the day and have a good power nap. Power naps are micro sleeping sessions that will help recharge your brain in a limited amount of time. However, you should be very careful that you don't let these power naps last for too long. Remember our discussion about sleep cycles? If you get into the deep sleep stage, you will find yourself feeling groggy and disoriented when you wake up from your nap. This is why it's better for your power naps to never be longer than 30 minutes. Also, avoid taking multiple naps in a day. One should be enough.

Force Yourself to Wake Up Earlier

One of the major reasons people struggle sleeping at night is that they wake up very late in the morning. Then, since they wake up late, they have a lot of energy that carries over into the later hours at night - and the cycle goes on and on. You can break that cycle by forcing yourself to just wake up early one morning. Don't hit the snooze button. Wake up, get off your bed, and do something productive. Make breakfast. Go for a run. Take a bath. Do whatever it takes to wake yourself up. You will find it a lot easier to go to sleep early at night if you wake up earlier too. Again, avoid pressing that snooze button.

Sleep in a Cool Room

Science has shown that sleeping in a room with lower temperatures will lead to better quality sleep. You are less likely to be woken up in the middle of the night when you are in a cooler sleeping environment. Also, it's easier for your heart rate to get lower when you sleep in colder temperatures. This means that your body is more prepared to slip into the deep sleep stage of your sleep cycle.

Engage in Cross-Training

Do cross-training. Do something that your body isn't used to. It's important that you introduce new stimuli to your training regimen so that your body is constantly being challenged in new paradigms. Over time, even as you increase load and volume with resistance training, your body will reach a plateau. Go out for a run every once in a while. Join a yoga class. These are all great ways to really approach your fitness more holistically. It will also keep you from getting bored by doing the same routine over and over again.

Do a Proper Warm-Up and Cool Down During Every Training Session

Don't just jump straight into a lifting session cold. If the workout says that you need to do five sets of five reps of deadlifts at 225 lbs, then you need to make sure that your body is prepared to handle that workload. The first thing that you need to do is warm up by breaking a sweat. Do some dynamic stretches that will activate your muscles, finetune your range of motion, and increase your heart rate. After that, do some light reps of deadlift first and gradually work your way up to your first set at 225 lbs. This is so you don't completely shock your body into a stressful condition. It will also help ensure that your muscles are ready for whatever you're going to put them through. Then, after a training session, make sure to do a proper cool down. Do some mobility work by doing a few static stretches or by foam rolling.

Devote at Least 10 Minutes Every Day to Mobility Work

It just takes ten minutes every day for you to improve your mobility over time. We've already talked about how mobility can help improve your performance at the gym and can help prevent any unwanted injuries. Just take ten minutes out of each day to focus on a specific muscle group for your mobility. Prioritize areas that are closer to your major joints, such as your shoulders, hips, knees, and ankles. For example, today, you could work on your hip area. So, you should be foam rolling your quads, hamstrings, and glutes. That whole process will only require ten minutes. The next day, you can focus on your shoulder by massaging your pectorals, scapula, lats, and delts. Again, target different muscle groups consistently and your mobility will develop over time.

Reduce the Amount of Stress in Your Life

Lastly, just reduce the overall amount of stress in your life. Don't sweat the small stuff. If possible, try engaging in meditation throughout various points of the day. Remember to always keep things in perspective. Stress is known to have some very ill effects on your body's natural processes. You are already stressed enough at the gym when you go through hard workouts. That should be enough. Any other unnecessary stress in your life should be avoided at all costs.

Chapter 5:

Training Your Muscles

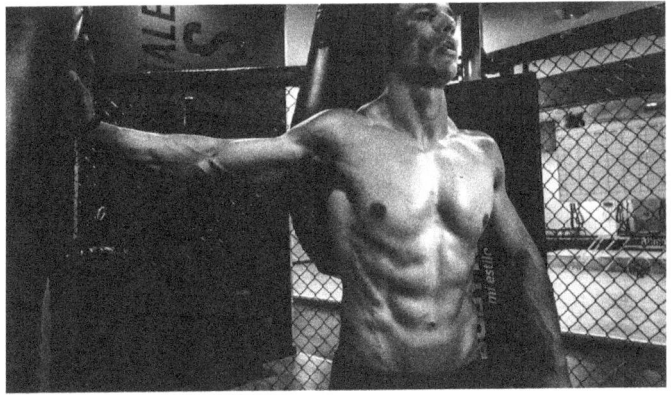

Now the time has come to talk about the exciting aspect of building your physique: training. There are some people who like to exercise and there are those who see it as a chore that they need to get over with. Regardless of how you view exercise in general, it's important that you have a very good relationship with whatever training regimen that you adopt for yourself. No two people should ever be given the exact same fitness and training regimen. There are a variety of variables that go into dictating what the perfect training pedagogy should be for you. However, it should be obvious that the more you enjoy and embrace your training, the more likely that you're going to be able to stick to it.

At the end of the day, that's the goal. You should be looking to build consistency with sustained efforts over a prolonged period if you want to see dramatic results. You can't expect significant progress in a short amount of time. This is why you need to adapt or build a training program that is designed for you to execute in the long term. Now, in order to do that, you need to orient yourself on the various movements that are involved in training your muscles. You have to start small. This chapter will help you learn all about the basic fundamentals of training specific muscle groups in order to stimulate growth and development. Once you have the knowledge on how to train specific muscle groups, you will also be taught about how you can string all of those different exercises together to create a cohesive and effective training program for yourself.

More than just learning how to make the most out of different exercises to stimulate muscle growth, it's also important that you know how to execute them properly. You must learn how to structure them into your program as well. If you perform a particular movement poorly, you could be doing significant and even irreparable damage to your muscles. If you're not structuring your program properly, then you might just be wasting all of the efforts that you're putting into the gym. It's imperative that you understand the nuances involved in structuring a strength training program so that you don't end up shooting yourself in the foot.

Before moving on, you should be proud of yourself for making it this far. Developing the resolve to pursue a greater body for yourself is something to celebrate. Unfortunately, not many are willing to put forth the time, effort, and commitment to pursue the best versions of themselves. By doing so, you are already separating yourself from the pack. You are a cut above the rest. Now, it's just important that you adopt the know-how that is necessary to get you to achieve your goals in the most efficient and effective ways possible. After all, none of this information is new or untested. This is knowledge that has been passed down by experts and enthusiasts over the years. Right now, muscle building is still a developing science and new breakthroughs and discoveries are being made every day. This is why it's important for you to continue to learn by reading books like these to help you stay safe and healthy as you train your body to its limits.

Compound vs Isolated Movements

Before we can get to the specific movements that are designed to stimulate muscle building, it's first important to identify the general classifications of these exercises. Generally, in any kind of exercise program, movements can be classified into one of two types: compound and isolated. Starting now, you should always be making it a point to prioritize compound movements as much as possible when adopting or creating a training plan. However, there should still be some room for isolated movements in your program as well. You will understand why as you learn more about the specific strengths and weaknesses of each movement category.

A compound movement is a type of exercise that requires the engagement or recruitment of multiple muscle groups found throughout various areas of the body. A classic example of such a movement is the deadlift. This requires the engagement of the core muscles, legs, and upper back. Another example of a compound movement is the pull-up which requires the engagement of the biceps, lats, and core. The reason that compound movements are much more beneficial for athletes is that they work multiple muscle groups in one go. This means that you're getting more bang for the buck with these movements. Also, compound movements tend to translate better into real-life strength. This means that they are more functional in nature and can help you get better with everyday tasks. For example, a deadlift can translate into helping you lift a big water jug or a piece of furniture off the floor. A pull-up can help you in situations where you might have to climb onto an elevated space using just your upper body. Aside from that, compound movements better develop your neurological fitness as well. Since you are working multiple muscle groups, your brain is getting its workout as well by trying to coordinate the proper function of these different muscle groups.

As you may have surmised, isolated movements are exercises that focus on single muscle groups at a time. They are designed to really target just one muscle group so that all of your attention is towards that specific area on your body. A classic example of an isolated movement is the bicep curl. A bicep curl, as its name implies, is a movement that only specifically targets the biceps. Obviously, the biggest disadvantage of an isolated movement is that you're not really getting the most bang for your buck. If you have a training plan that is composed purely of isolated movements, then it's going to take you much longer to complete a full body workout. However, that doesn't mean that isolated movements don't have a place in your training regimen. Isolated movements can be very effective for meeting specific goals such as correcting strength imbalances or weaknesses. This is a concept that is going to be discussed further in a later portion of this chapter.

Holistic Muscle Building

Now, it's time to talk about the importance of building your physique in a holistic manner. Too many times, people are guilty of avoiding working on their weaknesses and merely focusing on their strengths. This doesn't just happen in the realms of exercise and fitness. It happens way too often in various aspects of life. A writer who is skilled in writing romance will dare not practice writing fantasy novels. The martial artist who is good in boxing will be discouraged from engaging in wrestling drills. In bodybuilding, a person with strong legs is always going to prefer doing squats over pull-ups. As a result, they end up spending more time on the things that they are already good at just because they enjoy it more. This is the wrong approach to building your optimal physique.

An argument can be made that you should be spending more time on your weaknesses so that you have a more balanced approach to developing your body. If you know that you are leg-dominant, then devote more time and effort to working on your upper body. You don't want to end up having mammoth legs and toothpick arms, don't you? It's important that before you adopt a training plan, you assess your current fitness level first. Take a look at yourself in the mirror and perform an eye test. Does your body look proportional to you? Do your arms seem bigger than they should be? Is your waist a little pudgy? Are your legs smaller than the rest of your body? Once you determine what your strengths and weaknesses are, then you have a better idea of what you need to be working on when you make your training plan.

The Dangers of Muscle Imbalance

One thing that you must always be mindful of when you start your strength and resistance training is muscle imbalance. Too often, whether people are athletic or not, they go to visit therapists or chiropractors to help them with aches and pains in their body. A lot of the time, these aches and pains are brought about by muscle imbalances. Given that you're about to put your body through a stressful training regimen, you should expect that you would be more prone to developing muscle imbalances.

What is Muscle Imbalance?

To put it simply, a muscle imbalance is when one side of your joints exhibits considerably more strength than the opposing muscle on the other side of the joint. When talking in terms of physiology and biomechanics, this is not how your body should be structured or designed. When you have a muscle imbalance, this can be deemed as an abnormality that could potentially cause some serious complications in the way that you function biomechanically. When you have strength imbalances all over your body, one side could end up overcompensating for the other in order to cover that imbalance. This overcompensation could lead to potential injury and tissue damage.

What are the Symptoms of Muscle Imbalance?

Figuring out whether you have a muscle imbalance isn't always going to be so obvious, especially when you're doing it on your own. If you have a trainer who is watching you as you workout, they might have a better vantage point of spotting weaker areas in your body. However, if you're working out on your own, things might be a little more difficult as you have to engage in a high-level of self-assessment. Fortunately for you, there are ways in which you can test whether you have any existing muscle imbalances or not. Some of the most common symptoms of muscle imbalance include:

- lower back soreness/pain
- neck pain

- shoulder impingement
- knee pain
- rotator cuff tendonitis
- joint sprains
- tendonitis
- slipped discs
- muscle tears, etc.

Essentially, these kinds of injuries that seemingly pop out of the blue don't exist out of chance. They are there for a reason. You might be wondering what causes these little nagging aches and pains. Well, they could be caused by a number of possible reasons. But you should definitely be taking a look at any muscle imbalances that you might have

How Do You Address Muscle Imbalances?

Remember earlier when we talked about how compound movements are more efficient in helping you bulk up and get the body that you want? Well, that's still true. But we also talked about isolated movements and how they play a role in developing your overall strength as well. This is where they come in. The best way to correct muscle imbalances is to strengthen those weak muscles so that they are able to catch up to the rest of your body. Isolated movements that are designed to target specific muscles are great for correcting muscle imbalances. They are also great for providing accessory strength to your other compound movements which are inherently more complex.

For example, you might be doing a back squat and you notice that your legs are strong enough to push the weight up, but your core always gives in. You can then perform isolated movements that target specific muscles in your core to help you get better at a back squat. Another example of this is the pull-up. The pull up is a complex movement that recruits various muscle groups. There are some people who will find it difficult to perform a pull up properly because they are weaker in certain muscle areas. They might have enough strength in their lats to begin the ascent of a pull-up, but they might not have the bicep strength to finish it off. By doing bicep curls, an isolated movement, this can help correct the muscle imbalance so that the muscles recruited for a pull up will progress in a more unified manner.

Think of your muscles like a family. Every single muscle group is a member of that family and has some very specific roles to play when it comes to performing certain movements. When one member of the family is weak, then that compromises the performance of the entire family as a whole. Targeting your muscle imbalances is like finding the weakest link in your family and making sure that they aren't getting left behind. You always want to make sure that all of your muscle groups are progressing at a relatively proportional rate. As uncomfortable as it might be to confront your weaknesses, it's absolutely necessary that you address your muscle imbalances before they create any lasting negative impacts on your body.

Structuring Your Workout Plan

When it comes to structuring your workout plan, you have to keep in mind the various principles that we have discussed so far. To refresh, you need to prioritize compound movements so that your workouts and training sessions become more efficient. Next, you want to take a holistic approach to building muscle. This means that you never want to prioritize one muscle group over the other. Lastly, you want to avoid developing any muscle imbalances. This is why you need to create a workout plan that addresses all of your muscle groups and allows all of them the opportunity to grow and develop over time.

The first question that you might ask is how many times in a week should you be training. Well, the answer is going to be different from person to person. Again, it all depends on what your goals are and what your lifestyle is like. However, in general, you should shoot to have around four to five days a week of intense training if you're serious about building muscle. Again, it takes sheer will and consistency to achieve the body that you want. If it were easy, then everyone would be all chiseled up. Training sessions should typically be around an hour long. If you're efficient, you might be able to get things done in thirty minutes. It's all dependent on your level of fitness and how your body responds to training.

Push-Pull Movements

Aside from compound and isolation movements, we must also discuss push and pull movements. When talking about resistance training, your body is often doing either one or the other. It's either you're pushing against the force of gravity to lift a weight up or you're pulling against the force of gravity. A classic illustration of this would be a push-up and a pull-up. As you start choosing the movements that will make up your workout plan, you want to make sure that you are adding healthy doses of both push and pull exercises.

You can choose to approach this in either one of two ways. One is that you can dedicate one training session to exclusively push or pull movements and then alternate these sessions over the course of the week. For example, Mondays and Wednesdays can be dedicated to pushing movements while Tuesdays and Thursdays can be dedicated to pulling movements. Then, Fridays can be dedicated to a combination of both. However, another approach to structuring a push-pull training program is by incorporating both movements into every training session. For example, you might plan to perform six different exercises for Monday. Three of those exercises would be push movements and the other three would be pull movements. Then, you would carry this kind of exercise format throughout the week.

You might still be wondering why a push-pull movement or workout scheme would be beneficial to you. Well, ultimately, the answer can be summarized to the following reasons:

Offers Optimal Recovery

We've already talked about how rest and recovery are very important aspects of building muscle. The push-pull principle of training scheduling can help you structure your muscle recovery better. So, since you're splitting your training week into different segments (push and pull), then you're giving your muscles a chance to rest on days where they're not active. For example, if you are working on push movements on a Monday, then you are likely to engage muscle groups like quads, pecs, and deltoids. On Tuesday, if you are focusing on pull movements, then you are giving Monday's muscles a rest because you're focusing on other muscle groups like hamstrings, biceps, and lats.

Promotes Muscle Balance

By properly dividing a training plan between push and pull movements, it lessens the chance of developing a muscle imbalance. When you follow the push-pull principle of training, you have to make sure that you are getting equal doses of every kind of movement. If you have three exercises that are devoted to push-centric muscles, then you should also balance it out by having three exercises devoted to pull-centric muscles. This way, it's a lot easier for you to find that balance whenever you're drawing up your training schemes.

Prevents Injuries

This particular benefit of the push-pull philosophy of training is merely a byproduct of the previous two listed items. First off, if you are giving your body a chance to have ample recovery in between hard training sessions, then you are lessening the chances of your body giving up as a result of overtraining. Also, we talked earlier about how having a muscle imbalance could lead to someone being more prone to injury. Since the push-pull style of training lessens the chances of developing muscle imbalances, then it also negates any complications brought about by such a condition.

Provides Holistic Approach to Muscle Building

The push-pull method of training (paired with the integration of compound movements) can help you achieve a more holistic approach to muscle building. You would be able to target multiple muscle groups to make sure that every single area of the body is being given time and attention.

Saves Time

Lastly, it just makes your workout a lot more efficient. If you have a day job or a family, you don't want to be spending all of your time at the gym (unless you're a professional athlete). Ultimately, a push-pull philosophy can help simplify the way you structure your training so that you never have to rack your brain with thinking about what you're going to do on any given training day. So, aside from helping you be more efficient with your time spent at the gym, it also helps you be more efficient when you're plotting out your training schedule as well.

Upper Body Exercises

Your upper body includes all of the muscles that are found in your arms, upper back, chest, and shoulders. Functionally speaking, your arms are mostly responsible for lifting yourself up onto platforms or for moving heavy weight from point A to point B. There are a number of different upper body exercises that you can use for your training plan that are designed to target different muscle groups. Some of the most important compound exercises that you should integrate into your routine are going to be listed here.

Pull-Ups/Chin-Ups (Pull)

Pull-ups are a great pulling movement that helps build upper body strength. It's a movement that primarily targets your lat muscles. But it also helps strengthen your biceps and forearms, depending on the positioning of your grip. If you grip the bar with your palms facing towards you, it recruits your biceps more than your lats.

Variations: Supinated Ring Rows, Lateral Pull Downs

Push-Ups (Push)

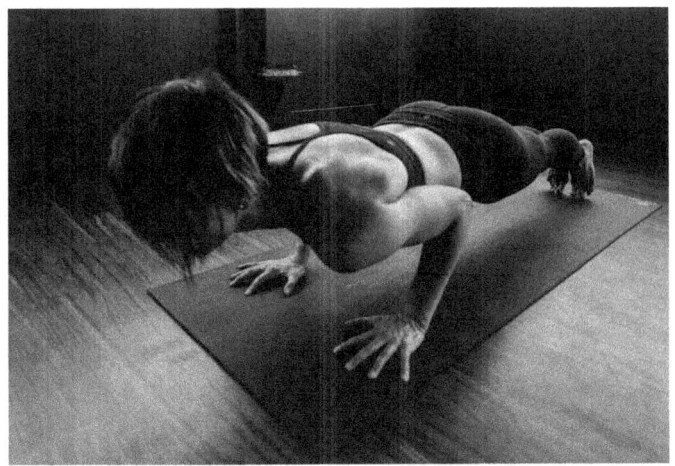

There are three major muscle groups that are being recruited to perform a proper push-up. For one, there are the pectoral or chest muscles. Then, there are the triceps, the muscles located at the back of your upper arm. Lastly, there is also the front of the shoulders or deltoids. The secondary muscle groups that are built by push-ups include the abdomen and the serratus anterior or wings. Like the pull-ups, you can change which muscles are being relied on depending on the positioning of your hands. A wider grip would place more emphasis on the chest while a closer grip places more emphasis on the triceps.

Variations: Push-Up on Ledge, Elevated Push-Up, Handstand Push-Up, Knee Push-Up, Dips

Bench Press (Push)

The bench press functions the same way as a push-up and recruits the same primary muscle groups. However, it places less emphasis on the core as you don't have to be propping your body up. Also, like the push-up, a closer grip recruits the triceps while a wider grip recruits the chest. This movement can be performed with either dumbbells or barbells.

Variations: Inclined Bench Press

Shoulder Press/Military Press (Push)

A military or shoulder press is a movement that can also be performed with barbells, dumbbells, or even kettlebells. It mostly targets the deltoids or the shoulders and has a secondary emphasis on the triceps. By extension, especially if performed in a standing position, the movement will also recruit the core and legs for added stability.

Rows (Pull)

A row is a movement that is often performed with dumbbells or kettlebells. However, there are variations that also allow for the use of barbells. The muscle groups that are mainly recruited when performing a row are the latissimus dorsi, trapezius, and rhomboid muscles. There is also a secondary emphasis on the biceps and forearms, depending on the positioning of the grip.

Variations: Bent-over Barbell Rows, Plank Rows

Special Exercise: Thrusters (Push)

The last upper-body exercise listed here is special because it is technically a full-body movement. The thruster can be performed with either a dumbbell, kettlebell, or barbell. It involves combining both a weighted squat and a military press all in one swift movement.

Core Exercises

Sure, it would feel and look great to have a six pack. But that really isn't the best part about having a strong core. When one talks about training the core, not a lot of people necessarily understand what muscles are involved in core training. Most of the time, they might think of the upper and lower abs, and maybe even the side obliques. However, your body's core muscles also include your glutes and lower back. All of these muscle groups are in charge of protecting and stabilizing your spine. Without a strong core, your spine would be very vulnerable and this could lead to some very serious injuries, especially when you're lifting heavy weights. You should always look to incorporate these basic core exercises into your training regimen.

Planks

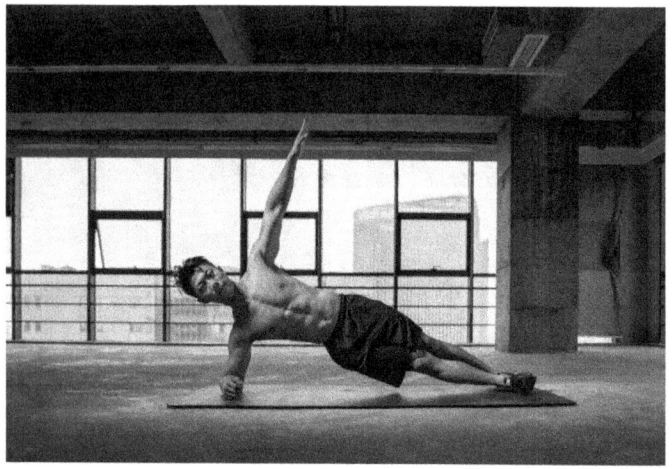

Many athletes and coaches will say that planks are the most efficient way to train your core. This is because the movement practically recruits every muscle group in your core region. It places a heavy emphasis on your frontal abdomen and your lower back. There is also a secondary emphasis on your gluteus maximus. There are also other variations of a plank that are more focused on the side obliques. Consequently, depending on how you position yourself in the plank, the movement can also improve shoulder stability.

Variations: Side Planks

L-Sits

The l-sit is one of the most complex core exercises because it requires a substantial amount of mobility and upper body strength to execute. Most people who are tight in the hips and hamstrings wouldn't be able to properly execute an l-sit due to their mobility issues. This is a movement that primarily relies on shoulder stability and pectoral strength for stabilization purposes. However, it requires a significant deal of abdominal and lower back strength paired with hip mobility in order to raise one's legs to a straight elevated position.

Variations: Hanging L-Sits, Seated L-Sits

Hanging Knee Raise

The hanging knee raise is a great core exercise that places a heavy emphasis on the frontal abdomen. However, it is also a great exercise for building grip strength and improving shoulder mobility. The general goal is to lift the legs by hinging at the hips and engaging the core.

Variations: Hanging Leg Raise, Toes to Bar

Back Extensions

Most core exercises tend to place a heavy emphasis on the frontal abdomen, side obliques, or the glutes. This is why it's important to incorporate back extensions into one's exercise routine as well because it targets the lower back, which is a part of the core muscle groups.

Sit-Ups

When you think of strengthening someone's abs, your mind might automatically picture someone doing a bunch of sit-ups. The primary muscle groups that are being recruited for a proper sit-up are the rectus abdominis, transverse abdominis, and obliques. Aside from that, sit-ups also help strengthen the lower back and hip flexors.

Variations: Crunches, Butterfly Sit-Ups, Weighted Sit-Ups

Lower Body Exercises

People love showing off their biceps, back muscles, or abs whenever they've been working hard at the gym. Although, you might not realize that some of the biggest muscles in your body can be found in the lower body. Think about how much you use your legs on a daily basis. Whenever you jump, walk, stand, run, or do anything that involves you moving around from one place to the next, you are using your lower body. You wouldn't be as mobile as you are now without your lower extremities. This is why it's important that you pay more attention to training your lower body as well. It isn't just about having the biggest biceps in town. As they say colloquially, don't skip leg day.

Squats (Push)

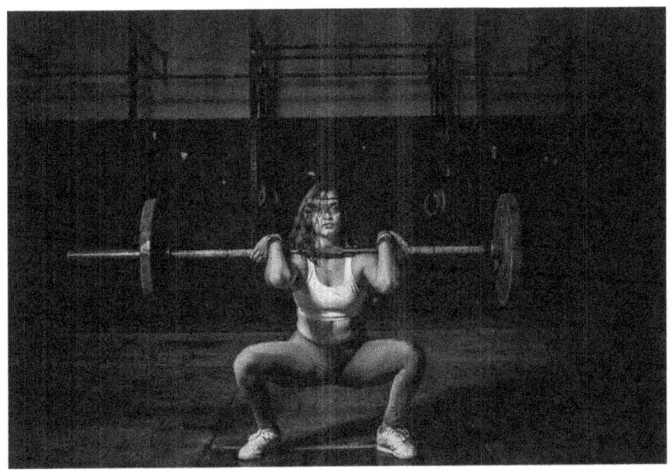

The squat is said to be one of the most important foundational movements that you could ever integrate into your workout routine. Having a strong squat translates to you having stronger legs that will serve as the foundation for whenever you stand, walk, jump, or run. The squat primarily recruits the quadriceps (front area of your leg), but it also has a secondary effect on your glutes, hamstrings, and calves as well.

Variations: Air Squat, Barbell Squat, Pistol Squat, Split Squat

Lunges (Push)

Lunges are like squats in terms of the muscle groups that they target. However, they offer a greater emphasis on single-leg engagement. This is an effective lower body exercise for addressing strength imbalances between both legs.

Variations: Walking Lunges, Reverse Lunges, Side Lunges

Deadlifts (Pull)

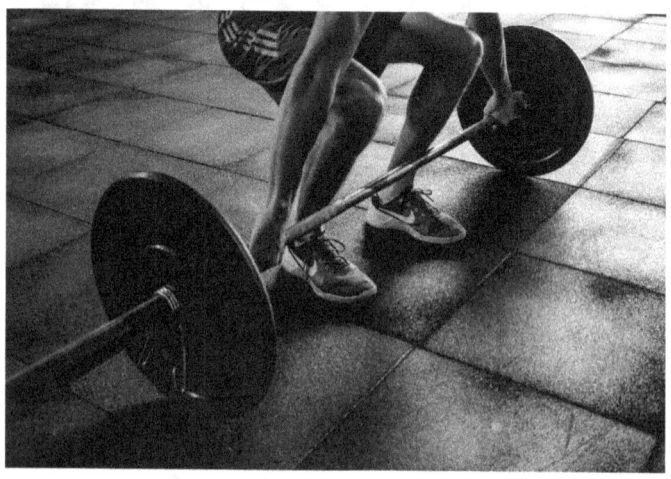

If the squat is considered to be one of the most important foundational movements in fitness, then so is the deadlift. Consider this as a *pull* variation of the squat, which is a *push* movement. The deadlift heavily targets the hamstrings, lower back, and glutes. However, it also requires substantial strength around the rest of the core muscles and the legs. Depending on how you position your feet, a deadlift can place heavier emphasis on a specific muscle group.

Variations: Stiff-legged Deadlift, Single-Leg Deadlift, Sumo Deadlift

Calf Raises (Push)

As its name implies, a calf raise is primarily focused on building up the calves. This is a very important exercise for those who are looking to build explosive strength that can translate into better running or jumping. Most leg exercises target the upper leg muscles like the quads and hamstrings. This is why it's important to integrate calf-dedicated exercises like the calf raise into one's bodybuilding routine.

Special Exercise: Cleans (Pull)

A clean is also technically a full-body exercise as it is a complex compound movement that recruits various muscle groups. The first phase of a clean is a deadlift that transitions into a powerful hip thrust paired with a violent shrug and pull from the arms into a strong front rack position. The first phase of a clean recruits the use of all the same muscle groups as a deadlift while the second phase of a clean recruits the same muscle groups as that of a row. The final phase or the catch position of a clean relies on pure core strength in order to stabilize the barbell.

Variations: Squat Clean, Power Clean, Muscle Clean, Dumbbell Clean

Special Note

Please remember that there are loads of different exercises and movements out there that can't be listed in this book for the purposes of practicality. Consider the movements listed here to be a list of capsule movements that you should have to serve as the foundation of your bodybuilding program. These are the foundational movements that will help you build that starting strength that you need to form good habits at the gym. Over time, as you become more experienced in this field, you will be exposed to more complex variations and modalities. Always feel free to explore these new areas of fitness. Be bold enough to introduce new movements and rep schemes into your training regimen. This is all a part of the process of testing your body's abilities and seeing just how much you're capable of.

Incorporating Cardio

If you're an ectomorph, then try to limit cardio as much as possible. Don't spend more than thirty minutes a week doing cardio. That wouldn't be beneficial to your current fitness goals just yet. If you want to improve your cardiovascular health, then just opt for shorter rest times in between sets while lifting. This will cause you to have a more elevated heart rate while training and this can also serve as a good exercise for your heart while doing resistance workouts.

If you're a mesomorph, you will need to do more cardio than an ectomorph, but not so much. Spend around thirty minutes to an hour every week that's dedicated to pure cardio work. Whether it be a jog on the treadmill or a spin class. It's important that you keep your heart healthy and that you do some activities that will help burn away the fat. You have a thriving metabolism and you don't have to worry so much about getting fat unless it's likely that you might be in a constant caloric surplus. Cardio can help make sure that you don't go overboard with your calories so that you don't get any unwanted fat.

If you're an endomorph, as expected, you're going to have to do the most cardio out of all the body types. Since you're most likely to gain the most pounds, you might have to do a little more work at the gym to burn off some extra calories. You can do 30 minutes of cardio around three to four times a week just to be on the safe side. Again, it doesn't always have to be running on the road or on a treadmill. You can do spin classes, rowers, ellipticals, and other cardio machines. You can also opt to play cardio-heavy sports like basketball, tennis, or football.

Using Supersets

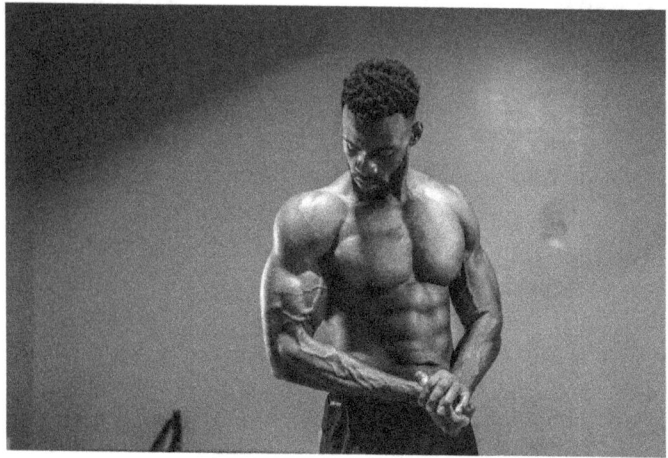

A superset is a common tactic that many lifters will use to introduce an added layer of difficulty and complexity to a workout. Aside from putting more stress on the body as a whole to produce better strength gains, it's also a more efficient way to go about a workout as it minimizes the amount of rest in between exercises. This way, athletes won't have to spend as much time as they need to at the gym.

The way that supersets work is that an athlete performs one set of a particular exercise and then quickly moves on to another set without any time for rest or recovery in between. The idea here is that it keeps the body constantly engaged and it trains the muscles to perform under stress. On top of that, it helps elevate the heart rate while performing resistance training exercises that usually don't have a cardiovascular component.

You can make use of the pull-push principle of training into your supersets by putting a push and pull movement against one another. For example, you might be using a squat as the first exercise in the superset. The squat is a push exercise. The next movement would be a row, which is a pull exercise. This is a great way to structure a superset because they offer different stimuli and both exercises recruit different muscle groups. So, while your lower body is recovering from the squats in the first set, you are still putting your body to work by using your upper body to perform the pull-ups.

Sample 1-Week Bodybuilding Program

Based on everything that you've been taught in this chapter so far, it's time for you to create or adopt a training scheme of your own. There are countless resources online that you can tap for ready-made training schemes. But it's also okay if you choose to make one on your own based on the knowledge that you have learned. It's also possible for you to find a ready-made program and tweak it a little bit so that it accommodates your own personal fitness level.

Here is a sample bodybuilding program that would be good for a week's worth of training. In this sample program, specific days are dedicated to push and pull movements with some days incorporating core training as well. You will also notice that during these exclusive push or pull days, there is a healthy balance between upper body and lower body exercises. Again, you want to make sure that you are taking a holistic approach to develop your fitness. It's important that you tackle different muscle groups. Also incorporated into this sample program are predetermined and mandatory recovery days. They are mandatory because that means that you have to rest on those days even though you might feel like you can go to the gym and lift. If you're feeling restless, then do some cross-training. Again, you shouldn't be training every single day. You need to give ample time for your body to recover in between long stretches of strength training. Feel free to take this sample program and adapt it to your own personal preferences.

Monday (Push + Core)

Push-Ups - 3 sets of 12 reps

Barbell Squats - 5 sets of 5 reps

Military Press - 4 sets of 10 reps

Calf Raises - 3 sets of 12 reps

Planks - 3 sets of 1-minute holds

Hanging Leg Raise - 3 sets of 15 reps

Tuesday (Pull)

Chin-Ups - 5 sets of 7 reps

Deadlifts - 5 sets of 5 reps

Barbell Rows - 3 sets of 15 reps

Cleans - 5 sets of 3 reps

Wednesday (Push)

Bench Press - 5 sets of 5 reps

Split Squats - 3 sets of 12 reps (each leg)

Dips - 3 sets of 10 reps

Lunges - 3 sets of 12 reps (each leg)

Thrusters - 3 sets of 15 reps

Thursday (Active Recovery)

Yoga, Swim, Run, Bike, or Mobility Drills

Friday (Pull + Core)

Pull-Ups (or Lateral Pull Down) - 5 sets of 5 reps

Dumbbell Rows - 3 sets of 12 reps

Deadlifts - 5 sets of 5 reps

Toes to Bar - 3 sets of 10 reps

Planks - 3 sets of 1-minute holds

Sit-Ups - 3 sets of 15 reps

Saturday (Active Recovery)

Yoga, Swim, Run, Bike, or Mobility Drills

Sunday (Rest)

Chapter 6:

Progressive Overload

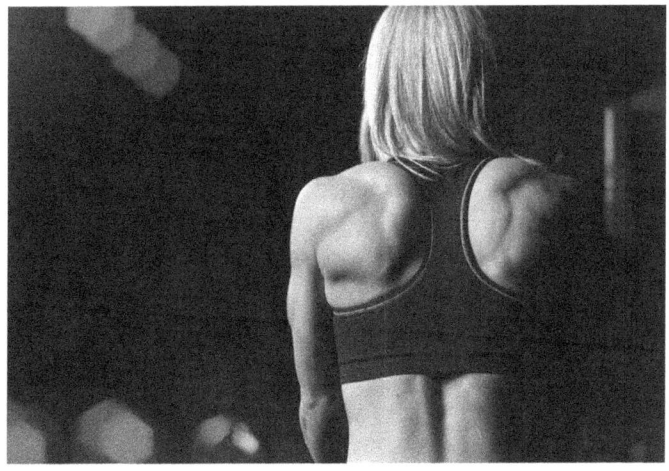

Let's say that you're done with finding a training program that works for you. You've done all of your research and analysis. You have already scoured the internet for many different workout programs and maybe you've consulted with licensed trainers or coaches to help you make a personalized program. That's great. But the job's not done. Learning and research do not stop. Just because you think you have a program that you're ready to start doesn't mean that you're going to be sticking to that program for the rest of your life. As you get better, fitter, and stronger, your workouts are going to feel a lot easier. When that happens, you know that it's time for a change.

One thing you have to know about the journey towards getting fit is that there is no destination. As cliche as it sounds, the journey is the destination. What this means is that the work is never really done. It doesn't matter how fit you become, there is always some work left to do. There is always going to be room for improvement. This is why you should be seeking progress, not perfection.

This chapter is going to help walk you through everything that you need to do AFTER you get started. Of course, getting started is a big step and you should always be proud of that. But it's not just about how you start. Results won't come just because you decide to get better with your fitness. Real results will only come if you continue to stick to the process and stay committed for the long haul.

What is Progressive Overload?

The whole principle of progressive overload centers around making your workouts more challenging over time. As you stay consistent with your training and workout regimen, your body is going to go through some amazing changes and transformations. You will find that things that you once found difficult are going to feel a lot easier and simpler to accomplish. However, while this might seem like good news, it's also going to be detrimental to your progress. The whole point of working out is challenging your muscles to the point of breakage so that there is ample space for growth and development. When there are fewer challenges, then there is also less room for growth.

Think of a first grade student who is just being introduced to basic math. They learn about addition and subtraction. They might even learn about multiplication and division. As they learn about these concepts, they are making substantial strides from when they first started. Over time, with enough practice, they get better at developing their mathematical skills to the point where these concepts no longer prove to be challenging. When that happens, their growth stops. This is why second grade students will then be introduced to the world of fractions and percentages. This is to add another layer of complexity and challenge to the students and by extension, it also expands their room for growth.

It's the same as when you workout. Progressive overload isn't a principle that is only applicable to strength training or resistance training. If you're a runner, you practice progressive overload by increasing the speed or distance of your runs. This is a concept that can be applied to so many different disciplines. It's all because it's one that promotes perpetual growth and development by continually introducing newer and more challenging stimuli.

How Does it Benefit Your Training?

One thing that you should expect to experience whenever you engage in resistance training is a plateau. The success that you get from working out is going to deliver some very remarkable results. However, this success that you gain isn't always going to be linear in its rate of growth. In fact, there is a good chance that the fitter you get, then the smaller your gains will end up being. Ultimately, it might even get to a point where your body will begin to plateau. This means that you are no longer getting any gains or experiencing any progress whatsoever.

The main reason for this plateau can often be attributed to your rate of effort. Obviously, the fitter you get, then the less effort is required of you to complete certain physical tasks. Pushing a 135-pound barbell overhead is going to be a lot more difficult at the start compared to when you're six or eight weeks into your training program. This is because you're getting fitter and the workouts are becoming easier. When your workouts get easier, you aren't really pushing your muscles to the point of breakage anymore. This is why progressive overload is the biggest tool that you can use to help combat whatever plateaus you might encounter on your road to fitness.

How Does Progressive Overload Work?

The concept of progressive overload is relatively simple. It's just a matter of you trying to find ways to make your workouts more challenging as you get fitter. Again, the fitter you get, the better you become at working out. This means that certain workouts that you did two or three weeks ago may no longer be as challenging now as when you first did them. So, you need to change these workouts up a bit in order to make sure that the stimulus still provides your body with a proper challenge. Now, how do you go about doing so? Well, there are three different approaches that you could take to introducing progressive overload into your training routine.

Increase Resistance

The first way to progressively overload yourself is to increase the level of resistance of your strength training. For example, let's say week one of the program had you deadlifting a barbell for five sets of five reps at 225 lbs. You repeat this cycle for maybe another week or two. Then, in the third or fourth week, you might find that these sets are a lot easier to accomplish and you're no longer challenged by it. You can make the exercise more challenging by increasing resistance or adding weight. In this case, you can up the weight to 235 lbs. This progressive overload is meant to adapt to your changing and improving level of fitness. Now, you might wonder about how much weight you should be adding. Well, it's going to be different for everyone as people tend to progress differently as well. However, a good rule of thumb to follow is that you should never look to increase the weight beyond 10% of what you were capable of lifting a week prior.

Increase Volume (Reps)

If you don't want to increase resistance, another way that you can go about introducing progressive overload is by increasing the volume of your workouts. If we stick to the same example of deadlifts at 225 lbs, you can still choose to keep the exercise at that weight as you get fitter. However, in order to progressively overload your system, you might want to increase the volume. So, try adding another set or a few extra reps for every set into your routine. Instead of five sets of five reps, maybe you can do six sets with the same rep scheme. You could also choose to stick to the same five sets, but with seven reps for each set now.

Increase the Rate of Work

Lastly, you could also opt to just increase your rate of work or productivity when you lift. Again, let's just stick to the same example of deadlifts at 225 lbs for the purposes of consistency. In the first week, it might have taken you around a full two or three minutes to recover in between each set. If you want to progressively overload yourself through increasing your rate of work, you can minimize the amount of rest that you take in between sets. By the fourth week, maybe your rest period in between sets would be around one minute to 90 seconds long instead of the two to three minutes you took when you first started. Even making this simple tweak can introduce a new stimulus to your body's muscular system and will offer the benefits of progressive overload.

Rules of Progressive Overload

By now, you should already have a good idea of what progressive overload is, why it's important, and how you're supposed to execute it. It's always good if you want to continue to introduce your body to new challenges, but you always have to be careful in doing so. By exposing your body to increasingly stressful environments, you have to make sure that you are keeping yourself safe and protected at all times. Progressive overload doesn't mean you going big whenever you're feeling confident. You still have to be methodical and tactical about it. Here are a few rules that you need to keep in mind when practicing progressive overload.

Always Start with Perfect Form

First of all, progressive overload should not even be an option for you if you're lifting with imperfect form. Again, if your form is bad, it doesn't matter how much weight you're lifting. You're doing it wrong and you're not going to get the gains that you want. Lifting with proper form means that you're engaging the proper muscle groups and that you're hitting all the right spots when it comes to your body's range of motion. If you can't perfect your form at lower weights or rep schemes, it wouldn't be wise for you to be progressing towards more challenging variations. There's no need to rush the process of progressive overload after all. Only move on when you're truly ready to do so.

Progressive Overload is Not a Linear Process

When you first start working out, you might think that you need to put the pressure on yourself to just keep on improving and improving at a rapid rate. In fact, you might create a schedule for yourself with regard to how much you should be lifting at a certain date. This is the wrong approach. You have to understand that your gains can't be scheduled. You shouldn't be giving yourself deadlines on how much weight you can lift. Progressive overload is something that you can only execute depending on what your body is capable of handling. It's not some kind of schedule that you NEED to adhere to in order for it to be effective. If your body is not capable of moving on from a particular level of resistance or volume, then stay at that level for a while.

Strength Gains Decrease Over Time and Increased Ability

Lastly, you have to expect that progressive overload is not going to become as rampant the older and more experienced you become in this field of fitness. When you're just starting out, it's very likely that you will experience significant jumps in your strength and abilities. This means that your progressive overload cycles might be a little more frequent. It's possible that you might be lifting significantly more weight in just a matter of one week. However, the more experienced and fitter you become, these strength gains become less and less frequent. There are some serious lifters out there who might even have to train a full year just to be able to gain 5 extra pounds on a single lift.

Chapter 7:

Final Tips to Remember

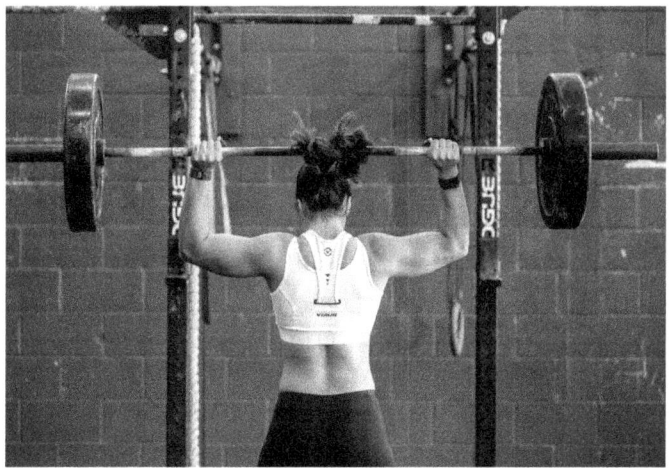

We're nearly reaching the end of the road here. You've come so far, but you still have far left to go. Fortunately, you know that you don't have to do everything on your own. Granted, this book might have been overwhelming to consume if you read it all at once. However, you will find that over time, with consistent practice, the knowledge in this book will become second nature to you. In fact, you might be able to write your own book on this topic one day. For now, just try to absorb little bits and pieces as much as you can and integrate these tidbits of knowledge into your daily training.

To conclude this book, here are a few key tips that you might want to keep to heart as you make your way through your fitness journey. Consider these tips to be the summary of everything that you've learned so far.

Don't Overtrain

Always make sure that you never overtrain. This means that you need to devote some time out of your training week to rest and recovery. Sure, you might think that doing more work will lead to more gains. That principle works only to a certain extent. Doing excessive work will not lead to gains. Rather, it will only lead to unwanted injuries that will sideline you and leave you worse off than when you started. Yes, you want to be giving it your best, but you don't want to overstretch yourself. In this case, it's better to work smarter than it is to work harder.

Leave Your Ego at the Door

One big mistake that amateur lifters or athletes make when they first start out is that they let their pride get to them. Sometimes, their pride will lead to them thinking that they're capable of lifting more weight than they can. What ends up happening? Injuries. Sometimes, their pride will have them believe that they are better or fitter than other people in the gym. This is the completely wrong mindset to have when approaching fitness. Your only goal at the gym every time you go there is to be better than the person that you were yesterday. Focus on that and the results will come.

Stay Consistent

Remember that old story about the tortoise and the hare? It's cool to be fast, but slow and steady wins the race. If you think that you can just go to the gym once or twice a week and give your maximum efforts for every session to get your desired results, then you would be mistaken. It would be a lot better for you to go to the gym multiple times a week and give small, but consistent efforts during every session. Eventually, these small efforts will add up to substantial gains that will only be given to you in the long run.

Don't Undereat

Even if you're an endomorph who is prone to gaining weight, it's important that you don't undereat. Of course, it should be obvious as to why an ectomorph shouldn't be undereating. Food is your friend, not your enemy. You need food in order to generate the fuel that is necessary for you to work hard at the gym. Without food, your muscles will not be able to grow and perform as efficiently as they should. It's all about moderation. You don't want to overeat, that's true, but it's just as important that you don't undereat.

Stay Hydrated

Always stay hydrated. Regardless if you're a serious athlete or not, you need water in order to survive. Whenever you put all of that hard work into your training, you are losing a lot of sweat in the process. You never want to end up feeling dehydrated as a result of your workout. Also, water is in charge of helping your body function properly, especially when it comes to processing nutrients from food. Water will help the protein synthesis process that is designed to help your muscle grow.

Prioritize Getting Quality Sleep

Sleep is a very undervalued resource that a lot of people take for granted. The amount of stress you put your body through as a bodybuilder is no joke. This is why you, more than most other people, need to devote more time to sleep. When you fall asleep at night, this is when your body is working double-time to revitalize and repair itself. Also, sleep is where you get a chance to regain your energy that will fuel you for another day of hard training.

Always Lift with Proper Form

Too many gym rats are guilty of this. Even people who have been working out for years can be guilty of this serious mistake. For the sake of completing a workout faster or for lifting heavier weight, some people will compromise their form in the process. This is a huge mistake because improper form while lifting (especially when the weights get heavy) can lead to serious life-threatening injuries. You would never want to attempt a PR back squat without bracing your core. This would be the quickest way to damage your spine and potentially paralyze you. Exercise in itself isn't dangerous and it's not something that you should fear. You just have to make sure that you are keeping yourself safe and protected by lifting with proper form every single time.

Only do the Recommended Amount of Cardio

The topic of cardio is one that has been exhausted numerous times in this book. Again, there is no definite volume or amount of cardio that all people should be devoting to every day or week. It all depends on your physiological makeup and your personal goals. However, as a general rule of thumb, if you're looking to build muscle, you want to focus more on resistance training while limiting any aerobic activities like running. This is especially true if you are an ectomorph who has a tendency to struggle with gaining weight. Doing a substantial amount of cardio might prove to be counterproductive to your goals.

Stop Measuring Your Success Against the Success of Others

The thing you have to remember about your fitness journey is that it's yours and yours alone. Unless you're talking about your trainer, coach, or therapist, your personal health and wellness goals are not of other peoples' business. The same is also true for you. If you see someone at the gym who is not excelling as rapidly as you, don't make fun of them. They are on their own fitness journey and it doesn't concern you. It's also the same when you see someone who you think is doing better than you. Just because they might seem more successful doesn't mean that you should invalidate whatever success you have. Be happy with your successes and leave it at that. Stop comparing yourself to others.

Don't Be Afraid of Supplements

Lastly, don't be afraid of supplements. No, whey protein is not a steroid. No, creatine is not a performance-enhancing drug. Supplements are filled with essential nutrients, the same that you would find in the food that you eat every day. However, supplements should only be seen as *supplementary* products to your diet. Ultimately, your diet should revolve around whole food like meats, vegetables, fruits, and grains. You should only use supplements whenever you feel like you need a few extra nutrients that you find difficult to source from natural food.

Conclusion

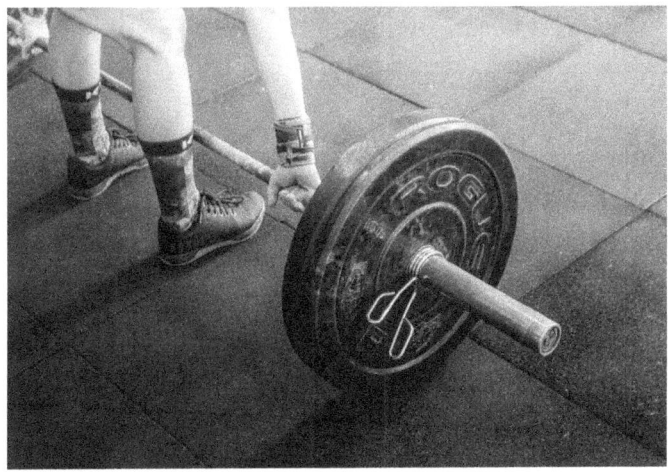

We're at the end now. Hopefully, this book will have inspired you to start strength training. At the very least, it should have added to your motivation to pursue a better version of yourself; the one that you deserve to be. Yes. You deserve to have the body that you want. Fitness is not a privilege or a luxury that is reserved only for those who are going to be blessed by it. Fitness is a right that you earn through sheer will, commitment, and hard work. Achieving fitness might not necessarily be easy, but it's always going to be possible. It doesn't matter what your background might be. Whether you had an athletic upbringing or not, you are still capable and worthy of pursuing and achieving your own personal fitness goals.

Too many people all over the world make the mistake of thinking that they don't have it in them to succeed. That's never the case. Improving one's fitness is a feat that is reachable and attainable for just about anyone. Even people with literal physical handicaps are capable of pursuing better versions of themselves. No, people don't lack the opportunities to become fitter. What they lack is the commitment and the willpower to actually pursue these goals.

You might have been guilty in the past of having a lot of excuses to not make the time for fitness. You were too busy. You felt like you didn't have the time. You didn't have enough money for a gym membership. These are excuses that all sorts of people have been using for the longest time now. Ultimately, what you have to realize about excuses is that you would never hear them from the people who genuinely want to make changes in their lives. This is because the people who are really willing to make these changes happen aren't going to be focusing on excuses. Rather, they focus on solutions. By reading this book, you are proving to yourself that you are shifting your focus towards the solution. You recognize that there is a problem and that there is room for improvement in your life. The fact that you're seeking out solutions is proof that you're ready to take that next big leap forward.

On your road to fitness, remember that you are going to encounter the occasional stumble. Success isn't going to come to you immediately and when it does, it isn't always going to be linear. You are going to have your fair share of ups and downs, just like in life. You might feel like you're taking two steps forward and one step back every so often. That's okay. That's perfectly normal. These kinds of slumps and setbacks are to be expected. They're not nearly as important as how you would respond to such occurrences whenever they take place.

Just remember that one of the most important traits that you need to develop here is persistence. There will always be a ton of excuses you can make for you to not get fit. There will be a variety of different factors out there that will discourage you from pursuing your dreams. You are bound to hit a few roadblocks that will just make you want to quit. But if you stay persistent enough, then none of these things will matter. They will merely be but a slight hiccup on your road to self-fulfillment.

As you go out and put forth the effort to get the body of your dreams, always stay confident in the fact that you are worthy of having such dreams, to begin with. Be proud of having the audacity to believe that you deserve to become a better version of yourself. This is not only beneficial to you, but also to the people who will see your work. You will serve as a light and inspiration to those who are afraid to start. Your spirit will become a source of empowerment and confidence for those who don't believe in themselves. That's also one of the best things about fitness. It's a community. Even though you might have your own individual goals and you mostly workout alone, you also know that there are other people out there who share similar struggles as you. There are also others who have dreams and goals that are just as big. Having that knowledge alone will give you a sense of solidarity from others in the fitness community to keep on going after what you want. And by actively participating in the community, you effectively do the same for the people around you as well.

References

Aceto, C. (2020, January 2). 10 essential nutrition tips for beginners. Muscle & Fitness. https://www.muscleandfitness.com/nutrition/gain-mass/top-10-beginner-nutrition-tips/

Behar, J. (2004, May 13). Rest and overtraining: What does this mean to bodybuilders? | bodybuilding.com. Bodybuilding.Com; Bodybuilding.com. https://www.bodybuilding.com/content/rest-and-overtraining-what-does-this-mean-to-bodybuilders.html

Bubnis, D. (2020, July 30). Progressive Overload: What It Is, Examples, and Tips. Healthline. https://www.healthline.com/health/progressive-overload

Butler, S. (n.d.). The Problem with Muscle Imbalances. Www.Thejoint.Com. Retrieved October 16, 2020, from https://www.thejoint.com/colorado/arvada/arvada-west-38021/188888-problem-with-muscle-imbalances

Chertoff, J. (2019, February 26). Muscular hypertrophy and your workout. Healthline; Healthline Media.

https://www.healthline.com/health/muscular-hypertrophy#how-to

Costello, J. (2017, October 12). 5 reasons why you should build muscle. ActiveSG. https://www.myactivesg.com/read/2017/10/5-reasons-why-you-should-build-muscle

Creicos, B. (2014, September). What is your body type? Take our test! Bodybuilding.Com; Bodybuilding.com. https://www.bodybuilding.com/fun/becker3.htm

de las Morenas, D. (n.d.). Bodybuilding Sleep: How to Maximize Muscle Growth While You Snooze | How to Beast. How to Beast. Retrieved October 16, 2020, from https://www.howtobeast.com/bodybuilding-sleep/

Ferruggia, J. (2013, November 14). How To Approach Cardio While Building Muscle. Muscle & Strength. https://www.muscleandstrength.com/articles/cardio-building-muscle

Fetters, K. A. (2018, March 23). 11 benefits of strength training that have nothing to do with muscle size. US News & World Report; U.S. News & World Report. https://health.usnews.com/wellness/fitness/articles/2018-03-23/11-benefits-of-strength-training-that-have-nothing-to-do-with-muscle-size

Frothingham, S. (2018, November 12). What is basal metabolic rate? Healthline. https://www.healthline.com/health/what-is-basal-metabolic-rate

Mason, A. (2018, May 15). Why simple push and pull workout routines are the best. Studio SWEAT OnDemand. https://www.studiosweatondemand.com/ssod-articles/schedule-best-simple-push-pull-workout-routine-plan/#:~:text=The%20primary%20muscles%20in%20a

Mazzo, L. (2018, April 2). Why core strength is so important (it has nothing to do with sculpting a six-pack). Shape; Shape. https://www.shape.com/fitness/tips/why-its-so-important-have-core-strength

T-Nation (2007, July 3). The push-pull workout. T-Nation. https://www.t-nation.com/workouts/push-pull-workout

Nilsson, N. (2003, October 20). Weights Or Cardio: What's It Going To Be? Bodybuilding.Com. https://www.bodybuilding.com/content/weights-or-cardio-whats-it-going-to-be.html

Quade, S. (2018, December 11). The importance of nutrition. Bodybuilding.Com; Bodybuilding.com. https://www.bodybuilding.com/fun/teen-quade3.htm

Ring, S. (2017, March 16). The 10 do's and don'ts of mobility. Bodybuilding.Com. https://www.bodybuilding.com/content/the-10-dos-and-donts-of-mobility.html

Tinsley, G. (2017, July 16). The 6 best supplements to gain muscle. Healthline; Healthline Media. https://www.healthline.com/nutrition/supplements-for-muscle-gain

Trinh, E. (2018, September 21). Push-Pull Training 101: Everything You Need to Know. Aaptiv. https://aaptiv.com/magazine/push-pull-training

Van De Walle, G. (2018, November 19). Bodybuilding meal plan: What to eat, what to avoid. Healthline. https://www.healthline.com/nutrition/bodybuilding-meal-plan#benefits

www.ingramcontent.com/pod-product-compliance
Lightning Source LLC
Chambersburg PA
CBHW072159100526
44589CB00015B/2288